Low Carb
for your cooking machine

The cookbook with 60 light and delicious recipes

Anna Lange

All advice in this book have been carefully considered and tested by the author and the publisher. A guarantee may nevertheless not be adopted. Any liability of the author or the publisher and its agents for personal injury, property damage and financial loss is follow legally excluded.

All rights, especially the rights of reproduction and distribution of the translation. No part of this publication may be reproduced in any form (by photocopying, microfilm or other method) without the written permission of the author or the publisher or electronically stored, processed, copied or distributed.

1st edition 2017
ISBN-13: 978-1548866792

TABLE OF CONTENT

Introduction 1

Why Low Carb? 3

Mix to enjoy 9

60 delicious recipes 12

Breakfast 13

Soups 30

Main dishes 44

Vegetarian main dishes 70

Smoothies 78

Desserts 91

Snacks 99

Concluding 106

Bonus 107

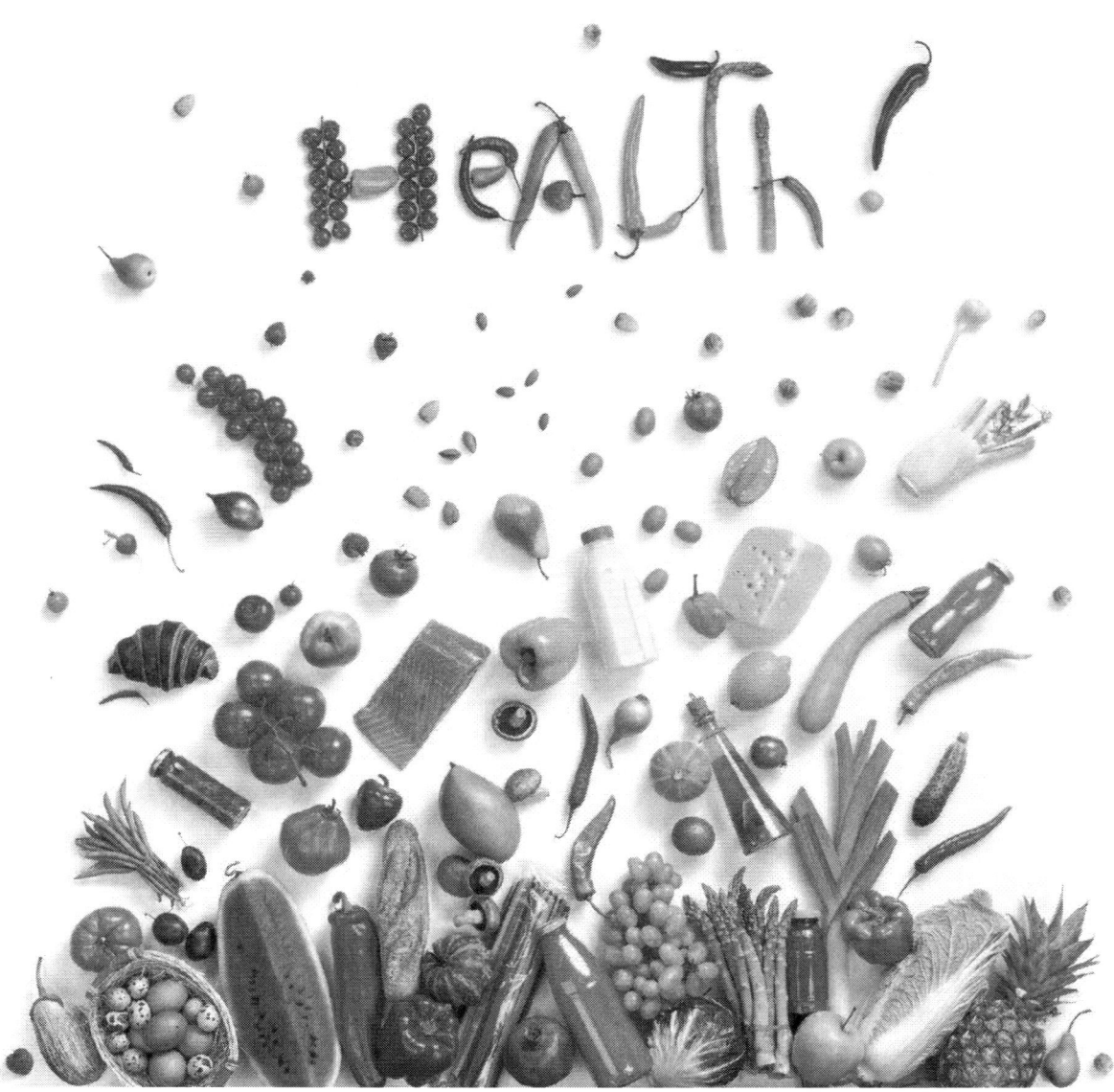

INTRODUCTION

A diet poor of carbohydrates is the first step on the way to a healthier lifestyle. It has a huge list of health promoting benefits to offer: weight loss, reduced blood glucose level, an elevated level of HDL cholesterol (the "good" cholesterol) and lower blood pressure are only some of them. Moreover, it spends significantly more energy, it avoids craving for sweets and leads to an improved level of triglycerides and insulin.

In this book you will find delicious recipes, all can be prepared easily and quickly with the well known mixing machine. This lets you not only save time and energy, it is also the perfect addition to your diet and your healthy lifestyle. No matter if in your job, while spending time with the family or on your holiday: A healthy diet is always important! The perfect time to start discovering these great recipes for your mixer is today.

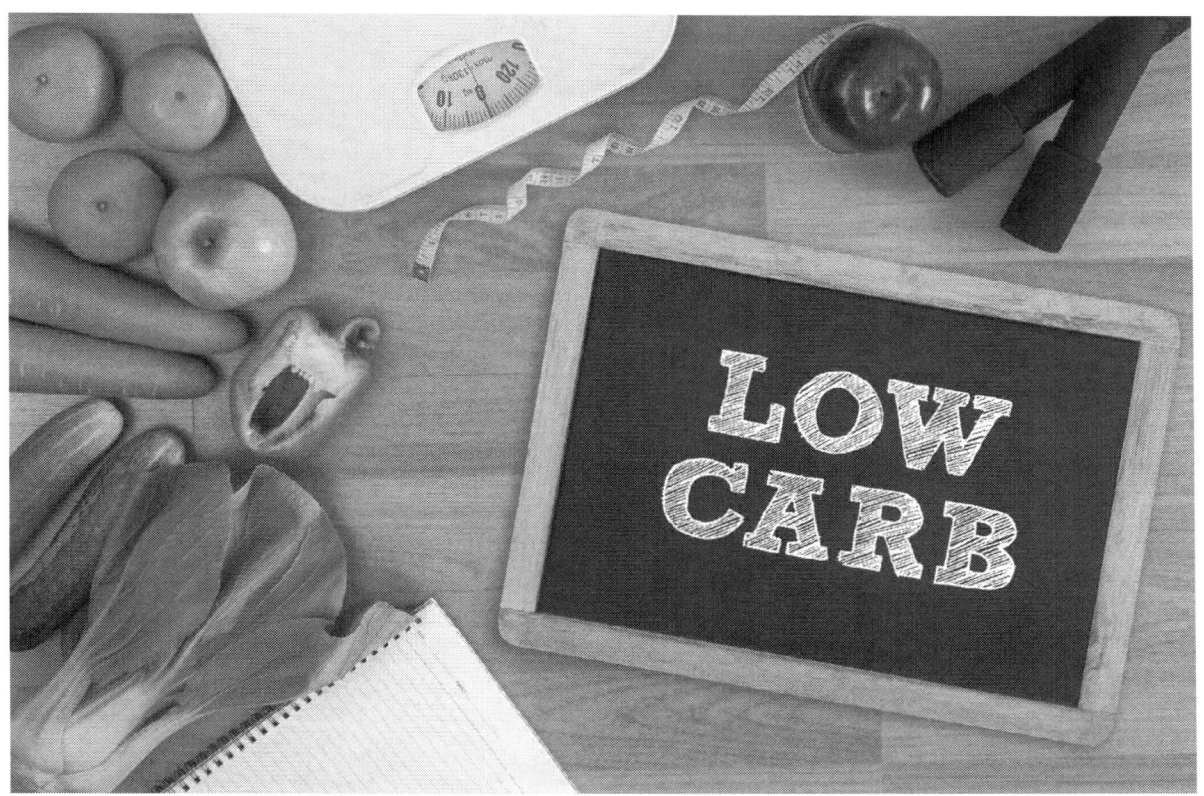

WHY LOW CARB?

Low Carb is constantly gaining popularity as more and more people are discovering its benefits. It helps you to achieve your desired weight while you are promoting your health. However, it has many more advantages to offer. Modern Western culture is full of acidic food, sugar, food additives, saturated fats, pesticides and hormones. Healthy ingredients are often lacking. Vegetables and fruits contain almost all the important vitamins, minerals, antioxidants and fiber your body needs to make you feel comfortable. In comparison calorie-rich and nutrient-poor food is often the reason for obesity and overweight.

Healthy eating is not only a question of quantity but of quality as well. Turning to a Low Carb diet, especially one that is rich in Omega-3 fatty acids with a lot of vegetables and less meat, helps you to detoxify and recreate your entire body. Your whole organism will recover and you will experience new strength or even feel vitalized for the first time at all. A diet containing lots of vegetables, beans, low-fat meat, fish, nuts, seeds, and fruits will give you all the essential vitamins and minerals your body needs constantly. Only one hand full of nuts contains your daily requirement of selenium and green vegetables and beans are just perfect sources of vitamin B, which is important for a healthy nervous system and brain. Achieving your desired weight or more physical energy is much more a question of what you eat than which kinds of pills or medicine to swallow.

Diabetes, insulin resistance and the Metabolic Syndrome all relate to a well known problem: The difficult to control blood glucose level. Diabetes and similar diseases are one of the major health problems in the western hemisphere. Patients suffering from diabetes are at a fourfold risk of dying from heart disease and also at fourfold risk of dementia. However, the results of scientific research show that diabetes can be treated nowadays, especially if it is diagnosed at an early stage. One conducted trial has shown that people suffering from Type-2 diabetes can recover only by changing their eating habits. Positive results were obtained in just one week.

A diet based on fruits can help you to control your blood glucose level, improve your metabolism and your health in general. Fibers slow down the absorbance of sugar into the blood, cause a feeling of being full and decrease cholesterol level. They also reduce the risk of developing certain types of cancer and cardiac disease. A healthy digestive system is ensured and a balanced intestinal flora is created.

No need to quit carbs completely

Many people starting a diet fail because they focus too much on starchy food. Bowls of pasta, rice or bread. Or even cookies. The problem is that their refined carbohydrates have a catastrophic effect on your glucose level and lead to huge variations of glucose and also insulin. With an increasing amount of glucose intake, insulin will send signals to your body affecting in the storing of fat, especially in the abdominal area as we all know it. Furthermore, it will create heartburn and a higher risk of developing insulin resistance in the long term.

A Low Carb diet is free of these refined sugars and starch. It instead focusses on "slower" carbohydrates (carbs being absorbed within a longer period of time). A good diet should contain a large variety of different vegetables. Starting a low glycemic and high fiber diet (containing slowly released carbs) you can be sure to avoid negative effects on your blood glucose level.

Healthy fats

Many people still associate fat with gaining weight only. But this is far away from the truth. While they have more calories than proteins and carbohydrates, the consumption of fat has a different effect on weight and metabolism. The right fats can even support your weight loss. Consuming more fat doesn´t only satisfy and stop your craving shortly, you will be full for a longer period of time. Healthy fats are Omega-3 and Omega-6, as well as Omega-9 monounsaturated fatty acids. Sources of these fats are Avocados, Cocoa and olive oil, nuts and seeds. Furthermore, integrating these fats will also help you to absorb fat solvent vitamins contained in sources such as tomatoes and carrots that can release their provitamin A to the body only under the presence of fat.

Recommendations for healthy food

- Nuts and seeds not only contain high amounts of healthy fats, they are also packed with vitamins, minerals, proteins and fiber. Their sources are food like macadamia nuts, almonds, peanuts, cashews, pecans, sun-flower seeds, sesame, hemp, chia seeds and pumpkins. Try to include at least two teaspoons of nuts rich of Omega-3 fatty acids in your daily diet.

- Eat leafy vegetables, very good promoters of Omega-3 fatty acids.

- Soy products contain Omega-3 fatty acids.

- Integrate monounsaturated fatty acids that are contained in olives, olive oil, avocados and macadamia nuts.

- Eat cocoa oil, cocoa milk and yoghurt or kefir.

- Choose cold-pressed oil, e.g. coconut oil, avocado oil, olive oil or nut oil. You can also add them to salads or use them for dips and smoothies. Avoid sunflower oil, soy or maize and vegetable oils as well as heated oils and margarine.

Recommendations for a balanced diet

Not to be frugal with:

At least half of your plate should be filled with a colorful variety of vegetables such as asparagus, aubergine, broccoli, cabbage, zucchini, cucumber, cauliflower, celery, dandelion, endive, fennel, garlic, ginger, artichoke, green beans, bell pepper, green cabbage, leek, mushrooms, onion, radish, celery, spinach, tomatoes or even watercress.

Recommended at high amount:

These high-fiber and high-protein food contain "slow" carbohydrates, avoiding huge jumps of blood insulin: Butter beans, black beans, cannelloni beans, soybeans, fish, chickpeas, lentils and pinto beans.

Food to avoid:

Why Low Carb?

Gluten-free grains and starch-containing food should be consumed only in small quantities. We recommend a maximum of one serving daily. Such food best to combine with your daily dinner are: Amaranth, buckwheat, gluten-free oatmeal, millet, quinoa, rice (whole grain), beetroot, carrots and sweet potatoes.

Dark berries such as blueberries, cherries, raspberries, currants and citrus fruits are known for their health supporting effect as well. They are low-glycemic food and thus can be recommended as an integral part of your diet.

Stone fruits such as nectarines, plums, apples and pears are good sources of fiber and release the "slow" carbohydrates into the blood. 1-2 servings of it are allowed daily.

To be recommended only to a limited measure:

Sugar contained in tropical fruits such as melons, grapes and pineapples should be consumed only in small quantities. Try to combine these with proteins and fat. Dried fruits are packed of sugar, so it is better to avoid them completely. Of course many recipes contain dates as ingredients. If you combine them with a protein source, the absorbing of sugar is slowed down into the blood and they can be consumed without having a guilty conscience.

Replace sugar with Xucker or sweetener. But be carefully here in dosing as well as sweetener should not be taken in too high amounts due to its different metabolism. Xylitol is a birch sugar and known for its laxative effect in larger quantities. If one is not used to this kind of sugar, the intake can result in bad times. We recommend to accustom slowly to these sugar replacements. Then they can be used quite easily. Another tip would be coconut blossom sugar or maple syrup. But again: Enjoy in moderation!

Food to avoid:

Gluten-containing seeds often cause allergies and can promote heartburn. So they can make it difficult for you to lose weight. Keep away from white flour, wheat, barley, rye and pasta. White sugar should be avoided! The same is agave nectar, this also applies to agave nectar, cane sugar, fruit juices or molasses.

10 Superfood, which you should include in your low carb diet:

- **Leafy vegetables** - This means green cabbage, chard and spinach. Perhaps you prefer green cabbage because it is rich in flavonoids, carotenoids, antioxidants, omega-3 fatty acids, dietary fiber, vitamin K, calcium, folic acid and iron. Spinach contains twice as much fiber as other vegetables and provides you with folic acid, vitamin B1, B2, B6, vitamin A, calcium, vitamin C, omega-3, iron, niacin, phosphorus and beta carotene. It will lower your blood pressure and help to avoid heart disease and bone loss.

- **Berries** - We recommend strawberries, raspberries, blueberries and goji berries. They contain fructose, but your body needs this sugar to remain healthy. Blueberries are good sources of antioxidants, vitamins A, C, E and K, zinc, calcium, manganese, lycopene, fiber, niacin, and help additionally against cardiovascular diseases.

- **Quinoa** - usually classified as grain, but is actually a seed, related to spinach and beetroot. There are many different colors in which Quinoa is sold. It has two big advantages: First, it is gluten-free and also a good source of protein what makes it a good choice for vegetarians. It is rich in iron and calcium as well as in mangan, magnesium, copper and fiber. Quinoa is really easy to cook and tastes delicious in a salad.

- **Amaranth** - another gluten-free cereal, that has a lot of protein, folic acid and vitamin B6. It is rich of fiber and grains that contain the amino acid lysine and regarding to the containing iron only topped by Quinoa. It has also been shown that it can help to reduce cholesterol. It is also the only known grain acting as a source of vitamin C.

- **Sweet potatoes** - promote vitamins and minerals. They are rich in vitamins A, C, D, B6 and packed of minerals, potassium, iron and magnesium. These potatoes should become a regular part of your diet.

- **Kiwi** - the delicious, slightly sour fruit shows that size does not matter. One big Kiwi covers your entire recommended daily amount of vitamin C. They are also rich in vitamins A and E. Eat at least a couple of them every week.

- **Chia and linseed** - the seeds are one of the best sources of omega-3 and omega-6. The only other way to get these fatty acids are fish oils. Chia seeds are a good source of protein and rich in calcium, potassium, fiber and vitamin B. Linseed inhibit the fight against cancer, the tumor growth and are proposed for the reduction of hormone metabolism.

- **Avocados** - a great source of unsaturated fats and also rich in potassium, folic acid and vitamin K and E. They are a great addition to sandwiches or salads.

- **Spirulina and Chlorella** - Spirulina is a cyanobacteria and one of the most nutritious food sources existing on the planet. It is a high-protein source that is rich in B vitamins and also helps to prevent anemia. It detoxifies, protects against radioactive damage and lowers cholesterol level. Similar to that is Chlorella, algae that has a detoxifying effect on the body as well. Combining these two algaes will have a huge improving effect on your health. Note: The taste needs a bit to get used to it at the beginning.

- **Almonds** - these nuts are full of vitamins, healthy fats and fiber. Because of their high content of fat, they are

Why Low Carb?

rich in calories and make them the perfect snack. Also to be combined with oatmeal, desserts and salads. So always have it with you!

The key to success

The key to success is a wide variety of food. Try to integrate all the different types of nutrients in your diet.

- **Proteins** - Protein forms our skin, hair and nails. and we essentially need it to stay healthy. And as already mentioned: Meat is not the only source of proteins. Spinach, kale, soy, beans, dried tomatoes, Brussels sprouts, broccoli and peas are the best of the most common and tastiest options. Fortunately, there is a large and manifold list to discover.

- **Calcium** - You should at least take up 1000mg of calcium daily, this is the equivalent of about three cups of milk or yogurt. Milk and yogurt are allowed in a vegetarian diet (not a vegan diet), but there are other great sources of calcium as well, such as green leafy vegetables, broccoli, beans, figs, sunflowers and corn. Vegetarians and vegans should integrate at least two servings of it in their daily diet to obtain the required intake of calcium.

- **Vitamin D** - vitamin D helps to absorb calcium and to transport it to bones and teeth. The human body produces the active form of vitamin D (in presence of sunlight) but consumption of food containing large amounts of vitamin D is recommended, especially during the winter months. Dairy products and eggs have many good sources of vitamin D.

- **Iron** - Iron is an essential element in the production of hemoglobin and blood cells, and therefore it prevents anemia. Sources are cereals, dried fruits, molasses, sesame, soy and dark leafy vegetables. Try to integrate food with high amounts of vitamin C in your diet as it is necessary to accommodate the iron into the body.

- **Vitamin B12** - This vitamin is found e.g. in dairy products and eggs. Vegetarians integrating dairy products and eggs in their diet should get a lot of this vitamin from these sources. Vegans can eventually consider adding a vitamin B-12 supplement to their diet.

Mix to enjoy

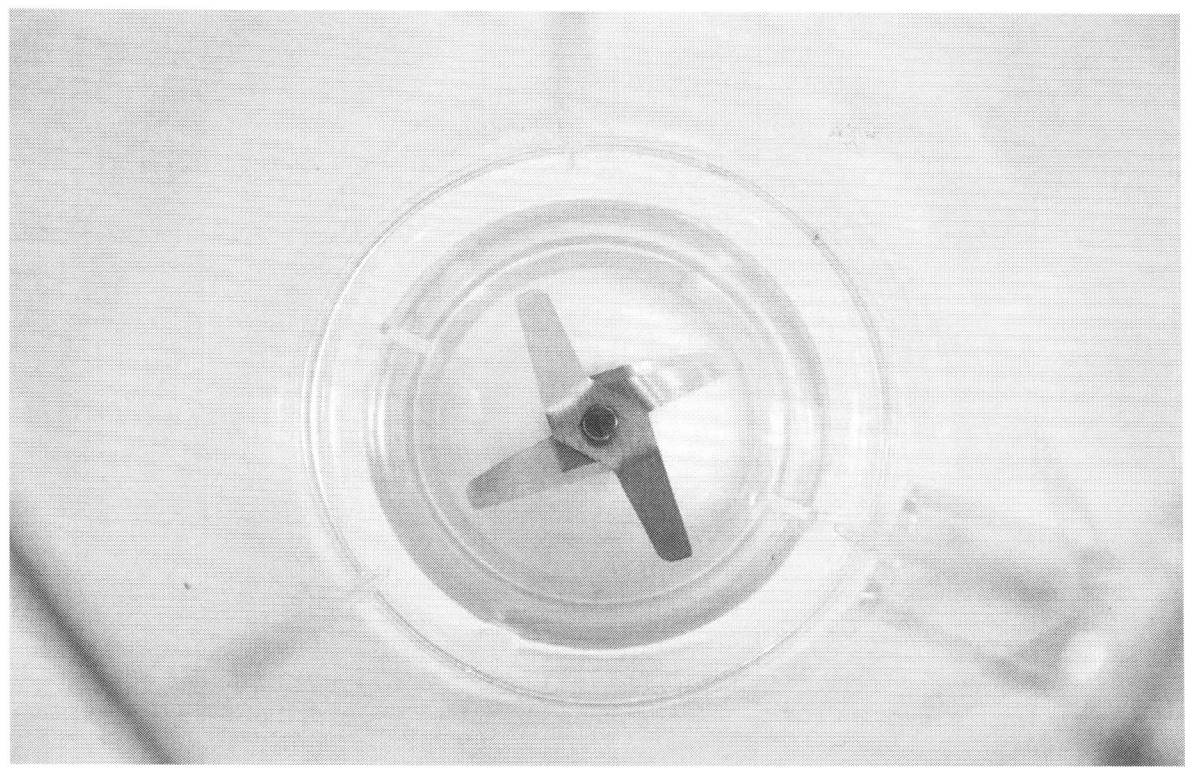

MIX TO ENJOY

The cooking machine is a high-tech kitchen gadget, combining a variety of different features in one single device, saving incredibly much space in your kitchen. The diameter of the device is no larger than a sheet of paper so it fits easily even in the smallest kitchen. Its functions are:

- **Steam cooking**: The cooking machine has an attachment called "Varoma" that gently cooks vegetables, fish and meat.

- **Emulsifying**: Prepare dressings for salads within seconds.

- **Kneading**: The cooking machine has a kneading function letting you save a lot of time when you are making doughs.

- **Cooking**: With the cooking machine you will be able to cook better than ever before. It gives you full

Mix to enjoy

control of temperature, time and intensity of stirring. You will be able to prepare almost any dish with just a single setting.

- **Controlled heating**: The cooker can be set at any temperature from 37°C to 120°C.

- **Grinding**: Make your own spice blend and grind anything simply by pressing a button. Nuts and seeds can be grinded as well.

- **Mixing**: A hand mixing device is no longer necessary. Make your own smoothies easily with this unique mixing device. Make sauces and dips within minutes easily with the touch of a button.

- **Stirring**: Simply adjust the stirring stage according to your recipe. The rest is done by the cooking machine. A very helpful feature as the ingredients of many recipes have to be stirred continuously.

- **Whipping**: Make your own whipped cream and whipped egg whites in an instant.

- **Weighing**: With the integrated scale all your ingredients can be measured quickly.

- **Crushing**: The sharp blades of the crusher will shred anything from cheese to chocolate, herbs, onions, garlic and more within seconds.

For whom it is suitable

This device is the perfect tool for everyone who enjoys baking and loves cooking with the goal to achieve a quick and good result. The recipes are easy to understand and a first success can be expected very soon. From cakes to goulash pan - anything is possible and prepared within just a few minutes.

Young families in particular will benefit from this Blender. Sometimes cooking can result in stress due to job, family and leisure activities on the route. The cooking machine is more than just any kind of compact kitchen helper. It is a tool for a healthier lifestyle that lets you still have enough time for all your other activities. So let´s begin!

60 delicious recipes

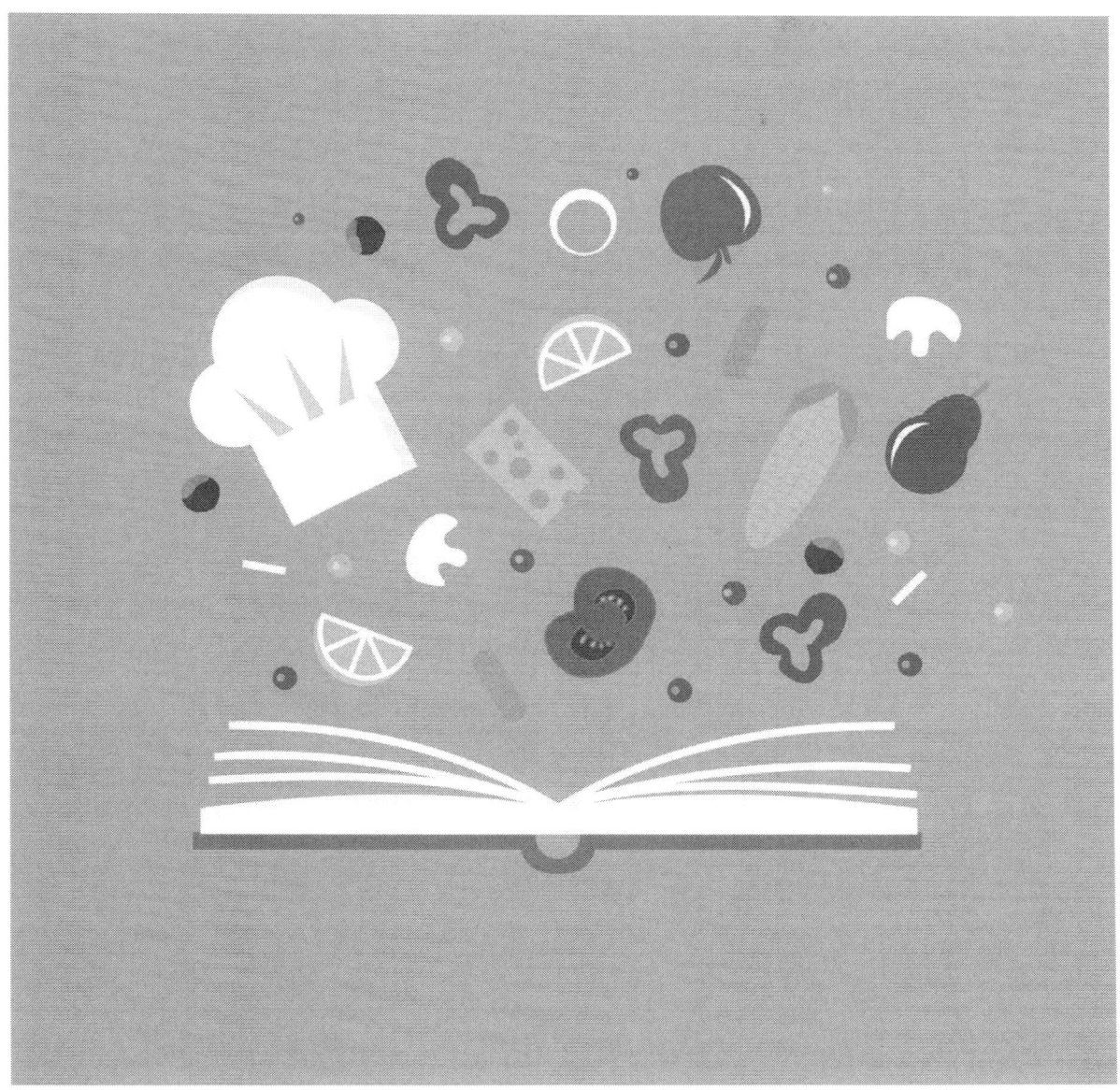

60 DELICIOUS RECIPES

Breakfast 13

Soups 30

Main dishes 44

Vegetarian main dishes 70

Smoothies 78

Desserts 91

Snacks 99

Breakfast

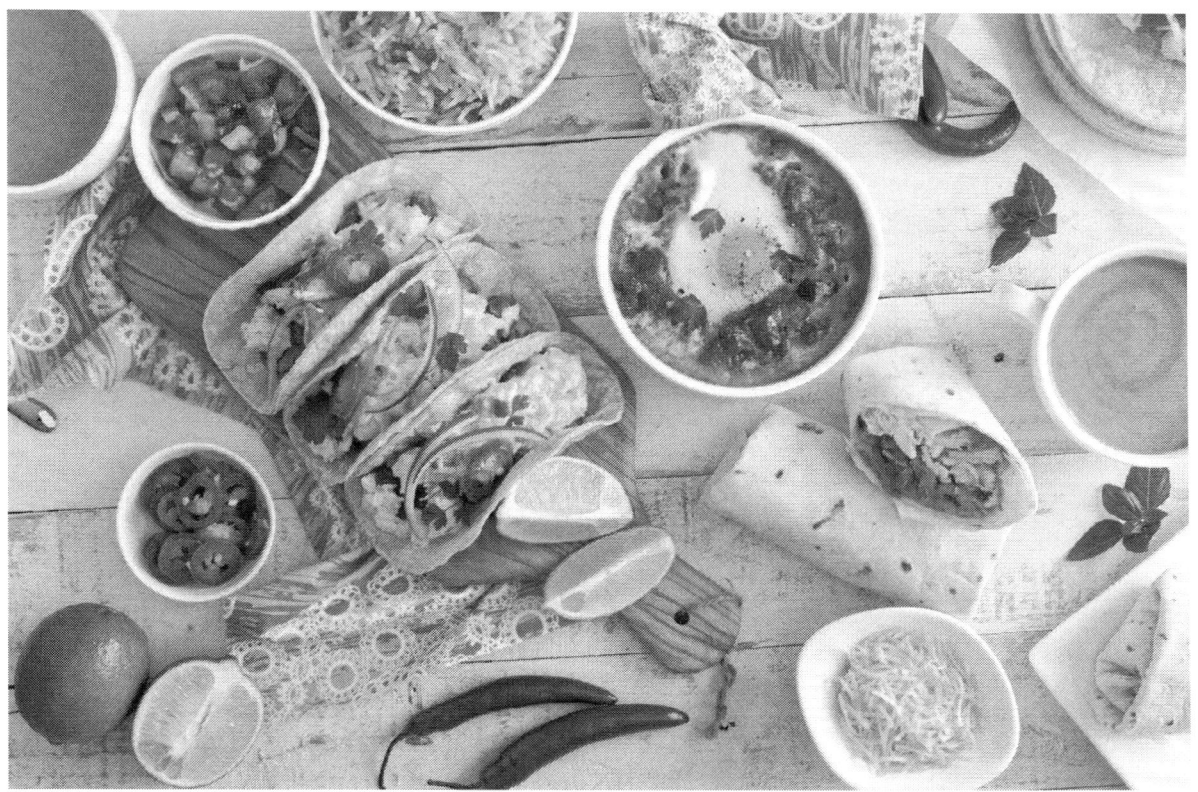

BREAKFAST

Mediterranean Tomato Bread 15

Linseed Bread 17

Walnut Bread 18

Almond bread 20

Olive and Parmesan Focaccia 21

Breakfast

Smoked Salmon Spread 23

Chives and Chili Spread 24

Oat Almond Puree with fruits 26

Egg Spread with olive 28

Low Carb Dip with feta 29

Breakfast

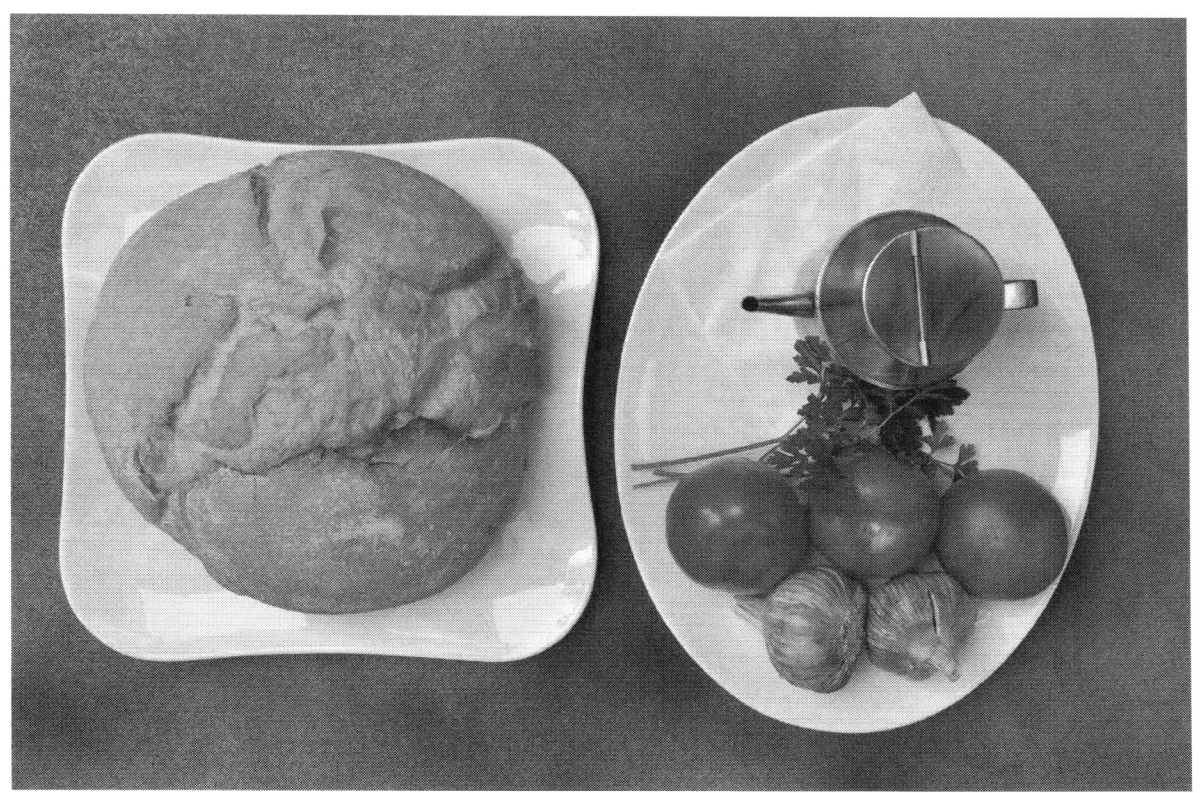

MEDITERRANEAN TOMATO BREAD

20 servings

Ingredients:

600g of linseed
60g of dried tomatoes
10 separated egg whites
4 eggs
12 teaspoons of olive oil
1 teaspoon of baking powder
2 stalks of oregano

2 stalks of thyme
Salt

Breakfast

Preparation:

Preheat oven to 200 degrees with upper and lower heat. Wash the herbs, dry shake and remove the starks. Add the linseed in the mix pot and then finely crush for about 10 seconds at stage 8. Then shred the tomatoes at level 5 for 4 seconds. Push them down in the mix pot with the spatula, then add the baking powder and the salt. Now mix at stage 3 for 5 seconds. Add the separated egg whites and the eggs and then start the kneading function. Let it run for 5 minutes.

Add 250ml of cold water and knead for another 2 minutes. Slowly add the olive oil while the kneading process continues. Cover a baking pan with parchment paper and fill the bread dough into the pan. Bake it at medium heat for 40 minutes. Let it cool for 10 minutes, then take the bread out of the baking pan and let it cool down completely.

KCAL	PRO	CAR	FAT
233	10g	2g	18g

LINSEED BREAD

20 servings

Ingredients:

600g of linseed
10 separated egg whites
4 eggs
6 teaspoons of olive oil
6 teaspoons of rapeseed oil
1 teaspoon of baking powder
Salt

Preparation:

Preheat oven to 200 degrees upper and lower heat. Chop the linseed at stage 8 until it is ground very finely. Add baking soda, salt, separated egg whites and the eggs and stir everything with the kneading function for another 5 minutes. Then add 250ml of cold water and mix for another 2 minutes. Slowly add olive oil and rapeseed oil while the kneading process continues.

Insert baking paper in a suitable form (e.g. a box shape mold) and pour the dough in. Bake it in the oven at medium heat for 40 minutes. Let everything cool down for 10 minutes and then take the bread out of the mold.

KCAL	PRO	CAR	FAT
227	10g	2g	18g

Breakfast

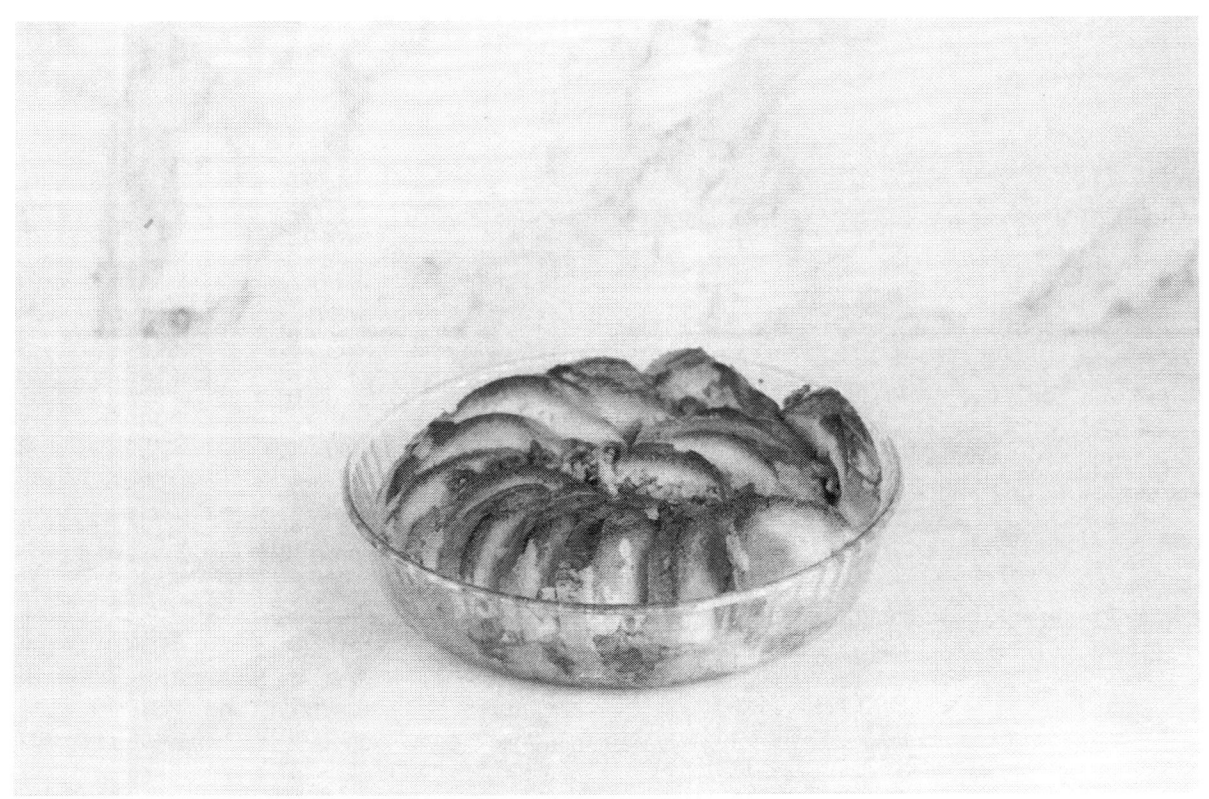

WALNUT BREAD

15 servings

Ingredients:

500g of linseed
125g of walnut flour
1 teaspoon of salt
10g of yeast
2 teaspoons of sweetener
½ teaspoon of olive oil

Preparation:

Put the linseed into the mix pot and add the salt. Crush it for 7 seconds at stage 8 until it is ground very finely. Now fill it into a separate bowl. Put the yeast together with 350 ml of lukewarm water in the mix pot. Add the sweetener. Now stir with the kneading function for 30 seconds. Add linseed and walnut flour and let the kneading function continue for another 5 minutes until you have a smooth dough. If your dough gets too dry, just add 1 or 2 teaspoons of water.

Shape the dough into a ball and place it into a bowl. Cover the bowl with a foil and let it rest in a warm place for an hour. If the volume of the dough has doubled, knead it once more again vigorously by hand. Cover a baking sheet with parchment paper and place the dough on it. Coat a large bowl with oil and place it over the dough. Now let the dough rest for another 45 minutes.

Now preheat oven to 250 degrees. Place a baking sheet filled with 450ml of water on the bottom rail of the oven. Place the baking sheet with the dough in the hot oven and bake it on the middle rack for 10 minutes. Then take the sheet with the water filled in out of the oven and reduce temperature down to 210 degrees. Bake for another 35 minutes, then open the door of the oven and continue baking for another 5 minutes with the door of the oven open. Now let it cool down on a rack.

KCAL	PRO	CAR	FAT
195	10g	8g	10g

Breakfast

ALMOND BREAD

15 servings

Ingredients:

500g of linseed
125g of almond flour
1 teaspoon of salt
10g of yeast
½ teaspoon of olive oil

Preparation:

Put the linseed into the mix pot. Add the salt and crush at stage 8 for 7 seconds. When the linseed is crushed finely, take it out of the cooking machine and put it into a separate bowl. Pour 350 ml lukewarm water in the mix pot and add the yeast. Now start the kneading function. Let it run for 5 minutes until you have a smooth dough. When it gets too dry, simply add 2 teaspoons of water.

Now form the dough into a ball and place it into a bowl, then cover the bowl with a foil. Let it rest in a warm place until the volume of the dough has doubled. Cover a baking sheet with parchment paper and put the dough on it. Cover a bowl with oil and place it over the dough. Now let it rest for 45 minutes. Preheat oven to 250 degrees.

Place a baking sheet filled with 450 ml of water on the bottom rail. Put the baking sheet with the dough on it in the hot oven and bake it for 10 minutes on the middle rail. Then take the sheet with the water added out of the oven and reduce temperature down to 210 degrees. Continue baking for another 35 minutes, then open the door of the oven and bake it for last 5 minutes.

KCAL	PRO	CAR	FAT
195	10g	8g	10g

Breakfast

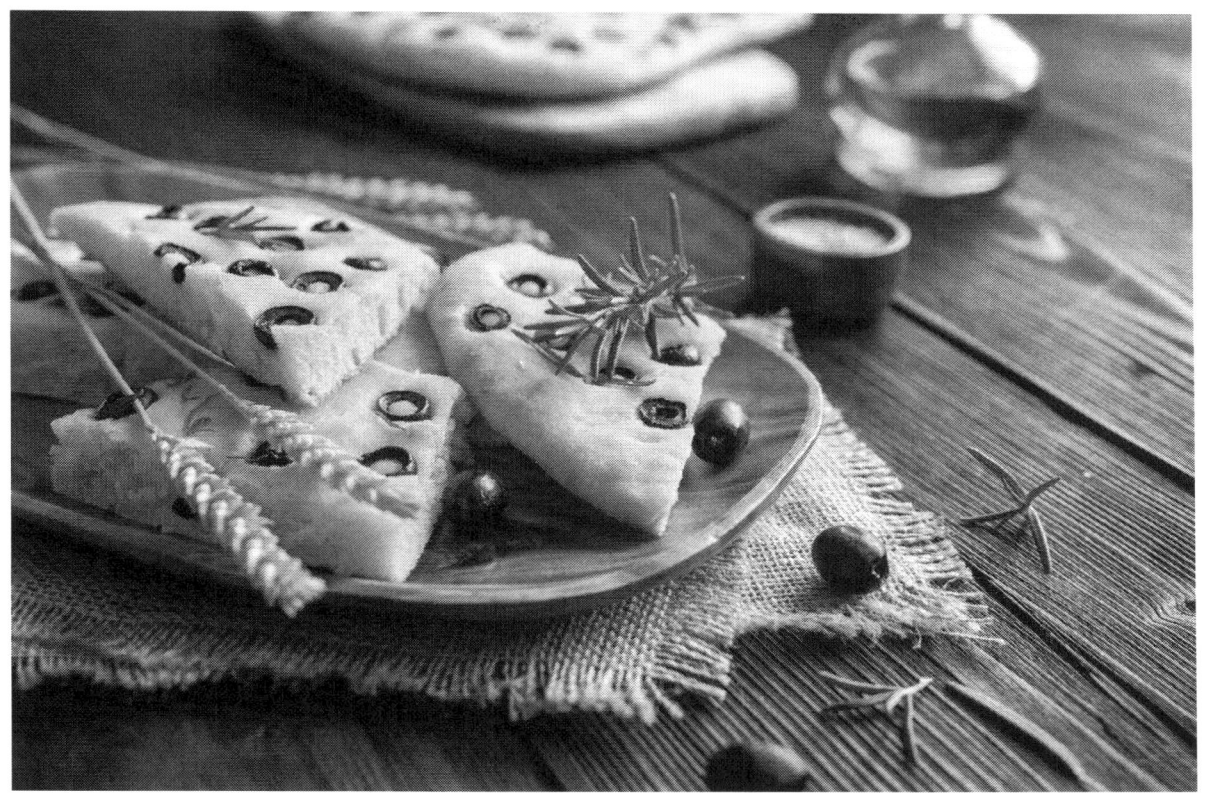

OLIVES AND PARMESAN FOCACCIA

For 1 Focaccia

Ingredients:

½ cup of linseed flour
1 egg
4 teaspoons of water
1 teaspoon of olive oil
1 teaspoon of toasted sesame seeds

¼ teaspoon of baking powder
¼ teaspoon of garlic salt
Pepper
15g of grated parmesan
40g of sliced olives

Breakfast

Preparation:

Whip the egg in the mix pot until it is foamy for about 4 minutes at stage 4. Add the remaining ingredients except the olives and stir. Then let the dough rest a few minutes. Spread the dough uniformly into a pan. Now sprinkle the sliced olives over it. Bake the Focaccia for 20 minutes at 180 degrees.

Nutritional values in total:

KCAL	PRO	CAR	FAT
1275	17g	6g	127g

Breakfast

SMOKED SALMON SPREAD

12 servings

Ingredients:

500g of smoked salmon
500g of creme fraiche
1 lemon
3 stalks of dill
Pepper (according to your taste)

Preparation:

Put the salmon into the mix pot and shred it at stage 8 for 7 seconds. Add the creme fraiche, then puree at stage 10 for 5 seconds. Squeeze out half a lemon and add the lemon juice. Wash the dill and remove the stalks. Then hack it coarsely. Add pepper according to your taste and puree at stage 10 for 4 seconds.

KCAL	PRO	CAR	FAT
210	9g	2g	18g

Breakfast

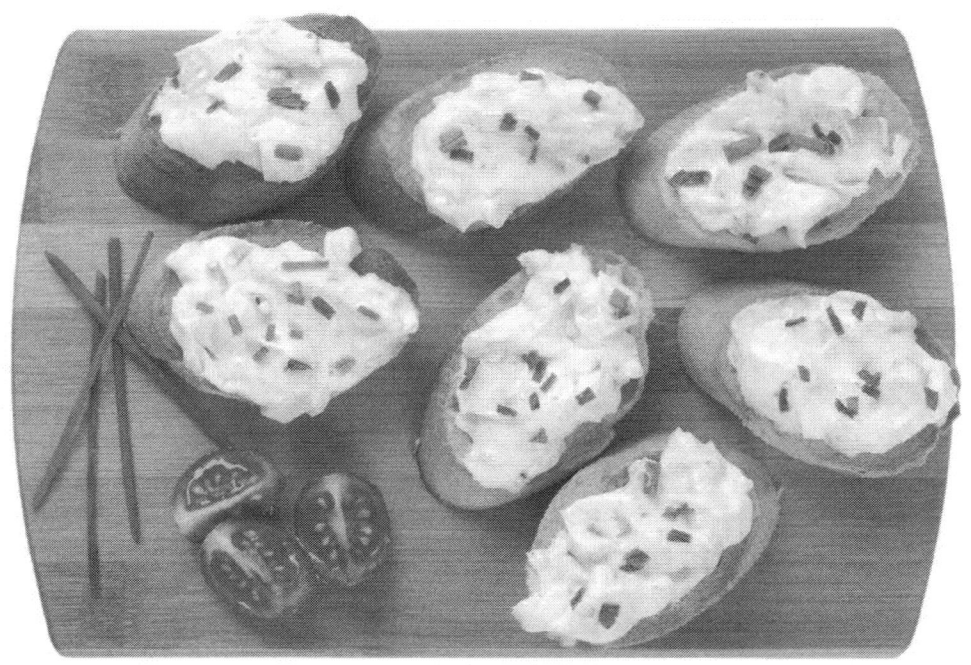

CHIVES-CHILI SPREAD

8 servings

Ingredients:

500g of creme fraiche

300g of sour cream

1 bunch of chives

2 green chilli peppers

Half a lime

1 clove of garlic

Salt, white pepper (according to your taste)

Preparation:

Wash the chives and chop it finely. You should remove the seeds from the chili peppers. The spread can get very sharp otherwise. Squeeze a lime and add the lime juice, then peel the garlic. Put garlic, lime juice, chili peppers and half of the sour cream in the mix pot and puree everything finely at stage 8 for 5 seconds. Then add the remaining creme fraiche, sour cream, chives and spices. Stir at level 3 for 8 seconds.

KCAL	PRO	CAR	FAT
270	3g	4g	26g

Breakfast

OAT ALMOND PUREE WITH FRUITS

1 serving

Ingredients:

60g of fresh raspberries

30g of almonds

15g of oat bran

1 teaspoon of sweetener or Xucker

130ml of low-fat milk

Preparation:

Grind the almonds finely in the cooking machine at stage 8 for about 10 seconds. Add oat bran, Xucker and milk. Alternatively, you can use a plant-based milk, such as oat milk or almond milk. Stir for about 8 minutes under heating at stage 2 (100 degrees). Put the almond paste in a small bowl and garnish it with the raspberries as desired.

KCAL	PRO	CAR	FAT
272	13g	13g	17g

Breakfast

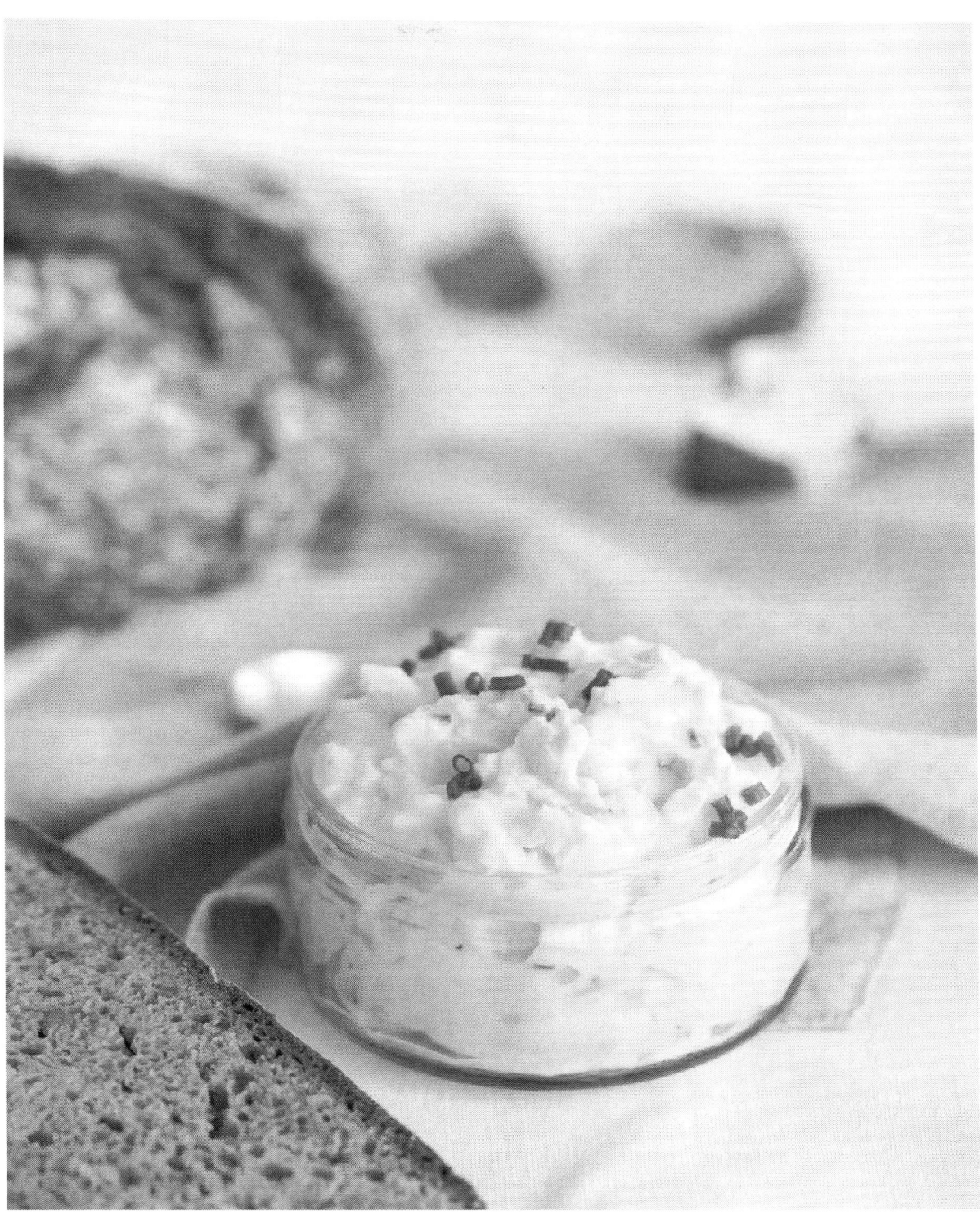

Breakfast

EGG SPREAD WITH OLIVES

2 servings

Ingredients:

4 eggs
60g of cottage cheese
30g of yoghurt
6 olives (green, seedless)
Ground lemon zest (from untreated lemon)
2 sprigs of tarragon
Salt, pepper, curry

Preparation:

Boil the eggs until they are hard. Dice the olives and chop the tarragon finely. Add cottage cheese and yogurt and mix for 5 seconds at stage 3. Add the remaining ingredients and stir for another 3 seconds at stage 2. Add salt, pepper and curry according to your taste.

Nutritional values per 100g:

KCAL	PRO	CAR	FAT
155	1g	2g	1g

Breakfast

LOW CARB DIP WITH FETA

1 serving

Ingredients:

50g of feta

130g of low-fat cottage cheese

Half a small cucumber

¼ teaspoon of lemon juice

¼ clove of garlic

Salt, pepper

Preparation:

Peel the cucumber and remove the seeds. Then cut it coarsely. Peel the garlic and chop the feta into coarse pieces. Put the cucumber and the garlic into the mix pot and then crush at stage 4 for 5 seconds. Add the remaining ingredients. Stir at stage 3. Add salt and pepper according to taste.

Nutritional values per 100g:

KCAL	PRO	CAR	FAT
221	25g	6g	9g

Soups

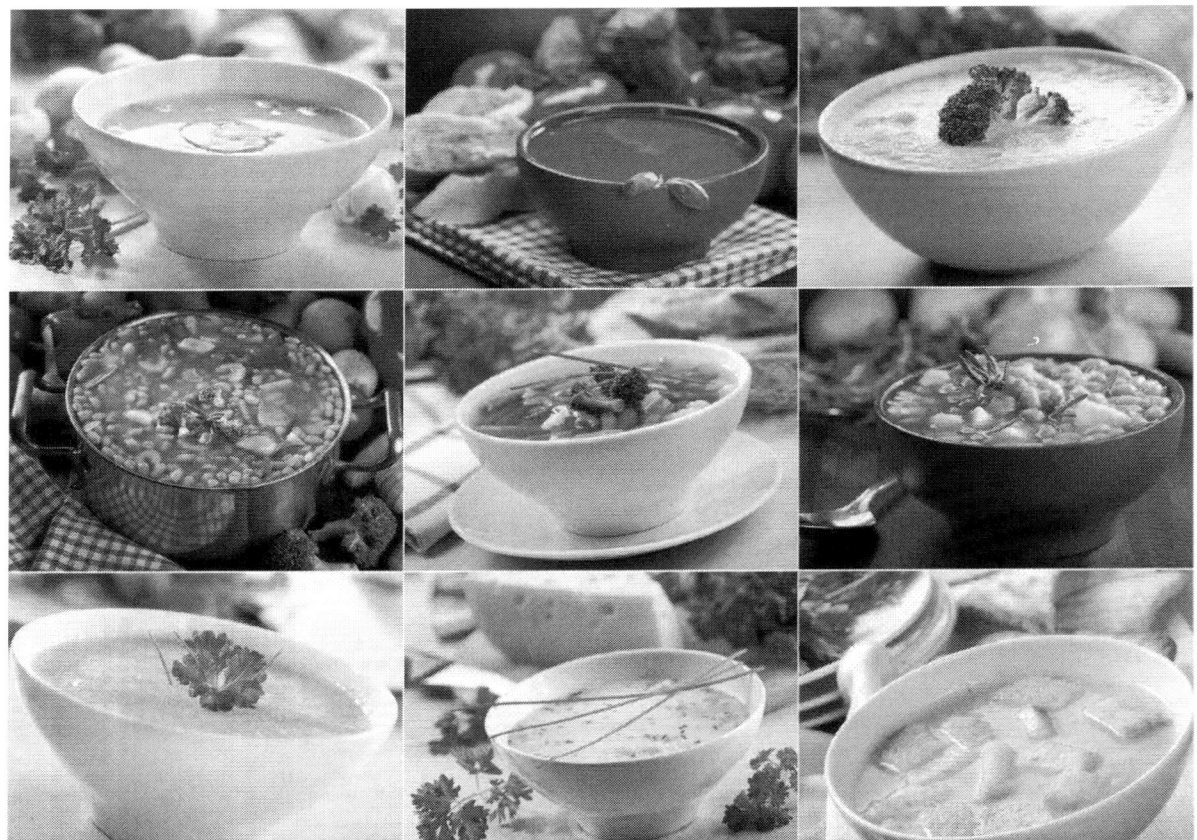

Spring stew with chicken 32

Hearty zucchini soup 34

Vegetable stew 35

Pumpkin soup 37

Broccoli cream soup 38

Soups

Coconut soup 40

Delicious leek cream soup 41

Low Carb cauliflower soup 43

Soups

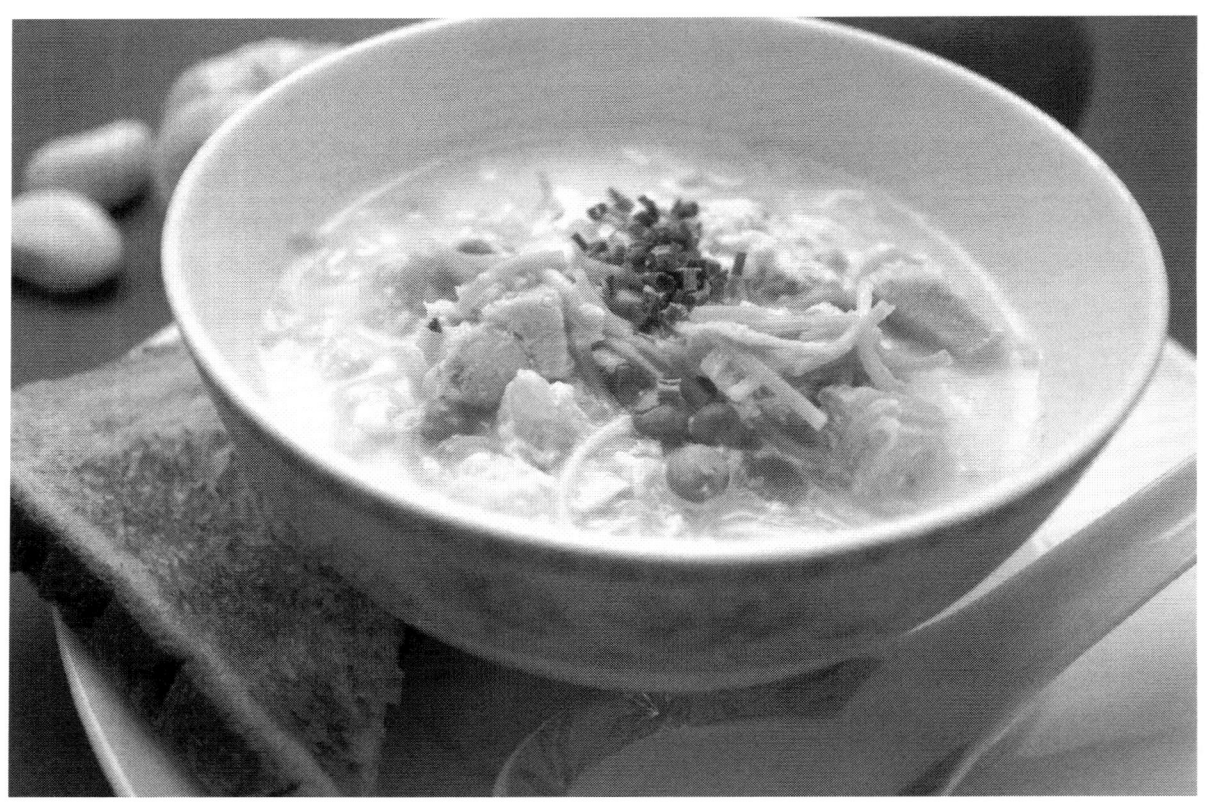

SPRING STEW WITH CHICKEN

2 servings

Ingredients:

300g of carrots

250g of broccoli

350g chicken breast

½ bunch of greens

Half an onion

1 teaspoon of sunflower oil

1 bay leaf

Salt, pepper, nutmeg

Preparation:

Peel the carrots, wash the broccoli and chop it into florets. Wash the chicken breast, pat dry and cut it into cubes. Brush the greens, then wash them. Peel the onion. Put carrots, greens and the peeled onion in the mix pot and shred at stage 7 for 5 seconds. Then add the oil and the vegetables and fry at stage 2 in left running mode for 3 minutes (100 degrees). Pour in 2l of water, add the chicken breast, the bay leaf, salt and pepper and simmer at 100 degrees at stage 2 in left running mode for another 50 minutes. 4 minutes before it is done add the broccoli and season with the spices.

KCAL	PRO	CAR	FAT
320	35g	14g	13g

Soups

HEARTY ZUCCHINI SOUP

1 serving

Ingredients:

200ml of vegetable broth

Zucchinis (225g)

5 small slices of zucchini (for the garnishing)

40g of cream

15g of butter

1 teaspoon of olive oil

1 pinch of nutmeg

Salt, pepper

Preparation:

Fry the zucchini with the butter for 7 minutes at stage 1 (100 degrees). Then add the vegetable broth and boil for another 15 minutes at stage 1 at 100 degrees. Puree the soup for 20 seconds at level 10. Add cream, pepper, salt, nutmeg and heat at stage 3 at 100 degrees. Serve the soup in a bowl.

Garnishing: Fry the zucchini slices gently in olive oil and spread over the soup.

Nutritional values per 100ml:

KCAL	PRO	CAR	FAT
520	8g	13g	46g

Soups

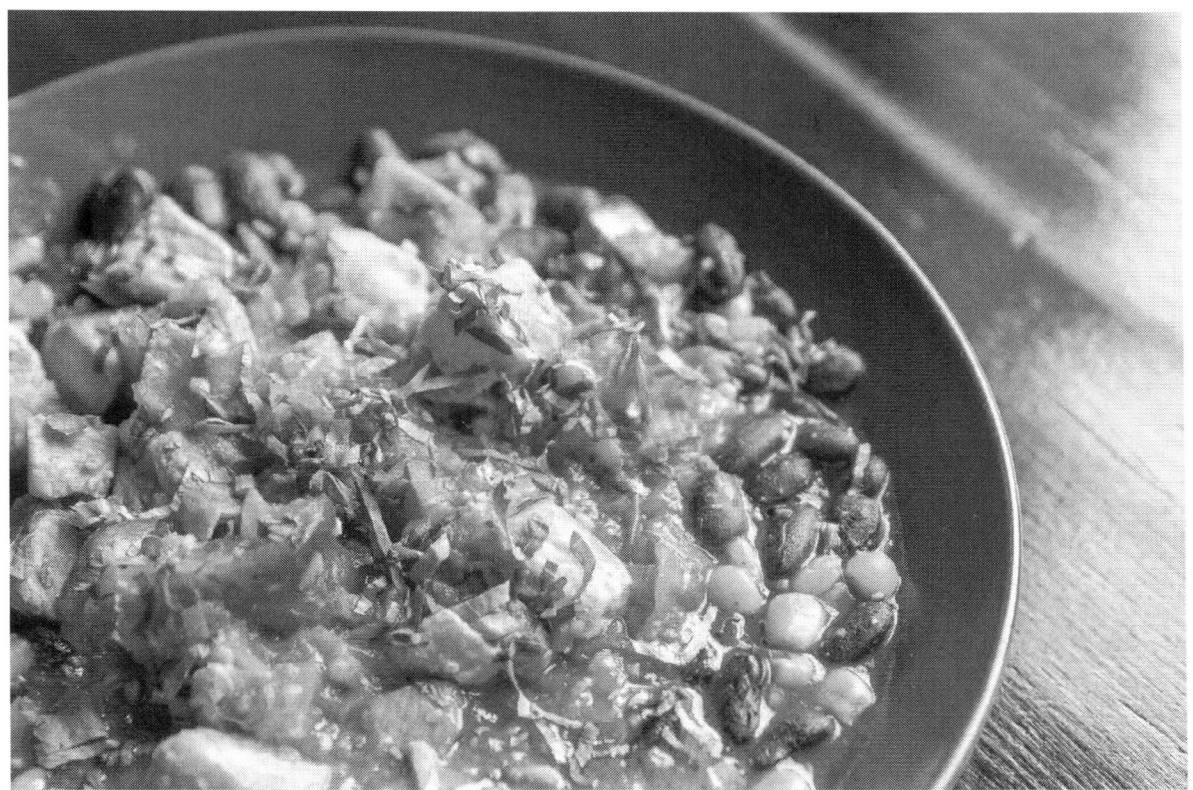

VEGETABLE STEW

2 servings

Ingredients:

½ eggplant

2 cloves of garlic

1 onion

250g pointed peppers

2 tomatoes

200g of chickpeas (canned)

600ml of vegetable broth

2 stalks of basil

2 teaspoons of olive oil

1 teaspoon of white wine

Salt, pepper

Soups

Preparation:

Wash the chickpeas in a sieve under running water and let them drain. Wash the chili peppers and cut them into rings. Wash the eggplant and the tomatoes and cut them into coarsely cubes. Peel the garlic and the onion, then quarter and put them in the mixing pot. Shred everything for 7 seconds at stage 5. Add the oil and steam at 100 degrees at stage 1 with the cooking machine. Add the eggplant and steam for another 3 minutes. Add the rest of the vegetables and pour the vegetable broth for 15 minutes at 90 degrees at stage 2 in left running mode. Spice up with salt and pepper. Garnishing: Wash the basil and remove leaves. Then spread them over the stew. Ready to serve!

KCAL	PRO	CAR	FAT
125	0g	18g	0g

Pumpkin Soup

2 servings

Ingredients:

350g Pumpkin

150ml of coconut milk

150ml vegetable broth

1 onion (middle sized)

2 cloves of garlic

1 teaspoon of oil

1 teaspoon of curry

Salt, chili

Preparation:

Peel the onion and the garlic. Quarter it and put it in the cooking machine. Then Chop for 7 seconds at stage 5. Add the oil and the curry and steam at 100 degrees at stage 1. Now Add the pumpkin. Pour everything with vegetable broth and coconut milk and continue cooking for another 20 minutes. Then puree on stage 8. Add salt according to your taste.

Nutritional values per 100ml:

KCAL	PRO	CAR	FAT
140	0g	18g	0g

Soups

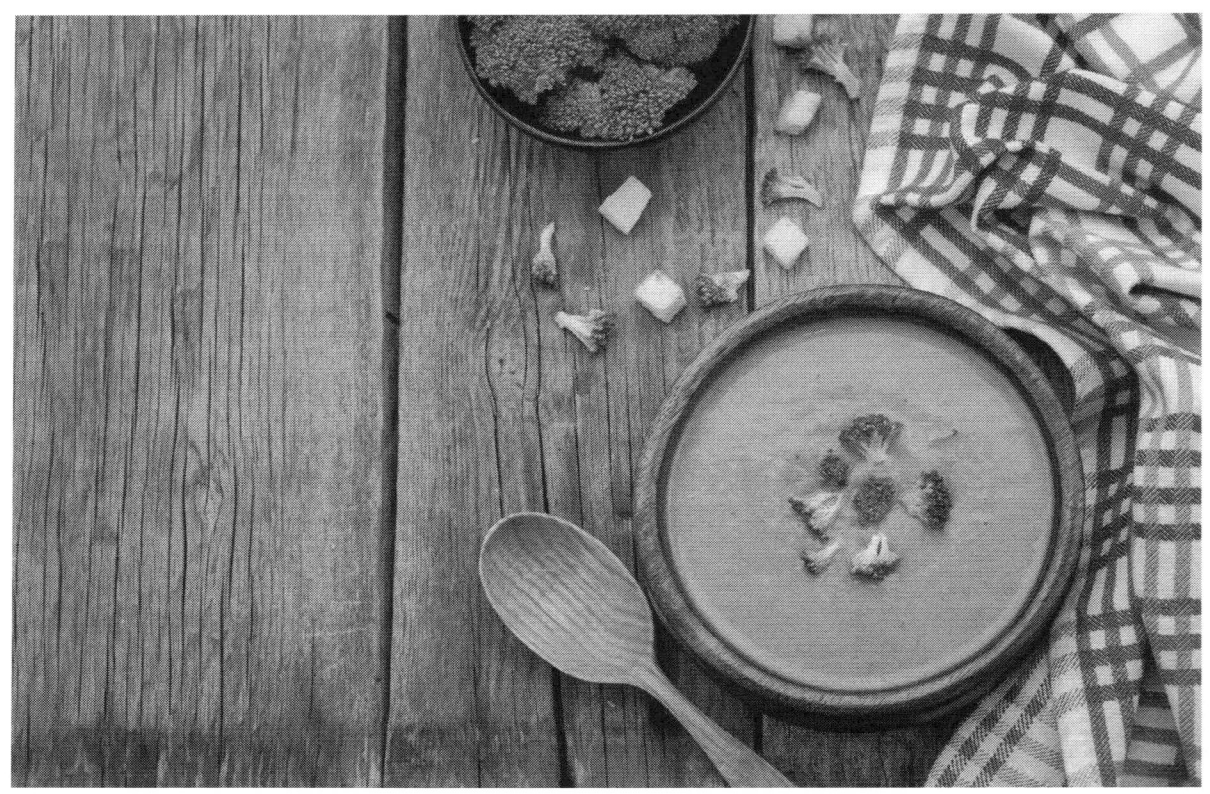

BROCCOLI CREAM SOUP

2 servings

Ingredients:

1 teaspoon of coconut oil

1 broccoli

1 small onion

1 clove of garlic

2 cups of water

100g of creme fraiche

½ lemon

Salt pepper

chili

Preparation:

Peel the onion and the garlic, then finely chop them. Put it in the mixing pot. Steam at stage 5 for 5 seconds. Then add the coconut oil. Cook for 2 minutes on Stage 1 of the Varoma application. Chop the broccoli coarsely and put it into the mixing pot. Steam a stage 1 for 5 minutes at 100 degrees. Pour in the water and add pepper and chili. Simmer for another 5 minutes. Sprinkle with fresh lemon juice.

KCAL	PRO	CAR	FAT
89	0g	5g	0g

Soups

COCONUT SOUP

2 servings

Ingredients:

400ml of coconut milk

300ml chicken broth

1 onion

1 clove of garlic

Half a small chilli pepper (red)

2 teaspoons of oil

1 small piece of ginger

1 tablespoon of curry

Preparation:

Peel the onion and the garlic, remove the cores from the chili peppers and put them in the mixing pot. Crush for 7 seconds at stage 5, then add the oil and cook at 100 ° C. Now add the curry and the ginger and steam briefly with the chicken broth, add the coconut milk and simmer for 10 minutes at 90 ° C. Now puree at stage 7.

KCAL	PRO	CAR	FAT
89	0g	5g	0g

Soups

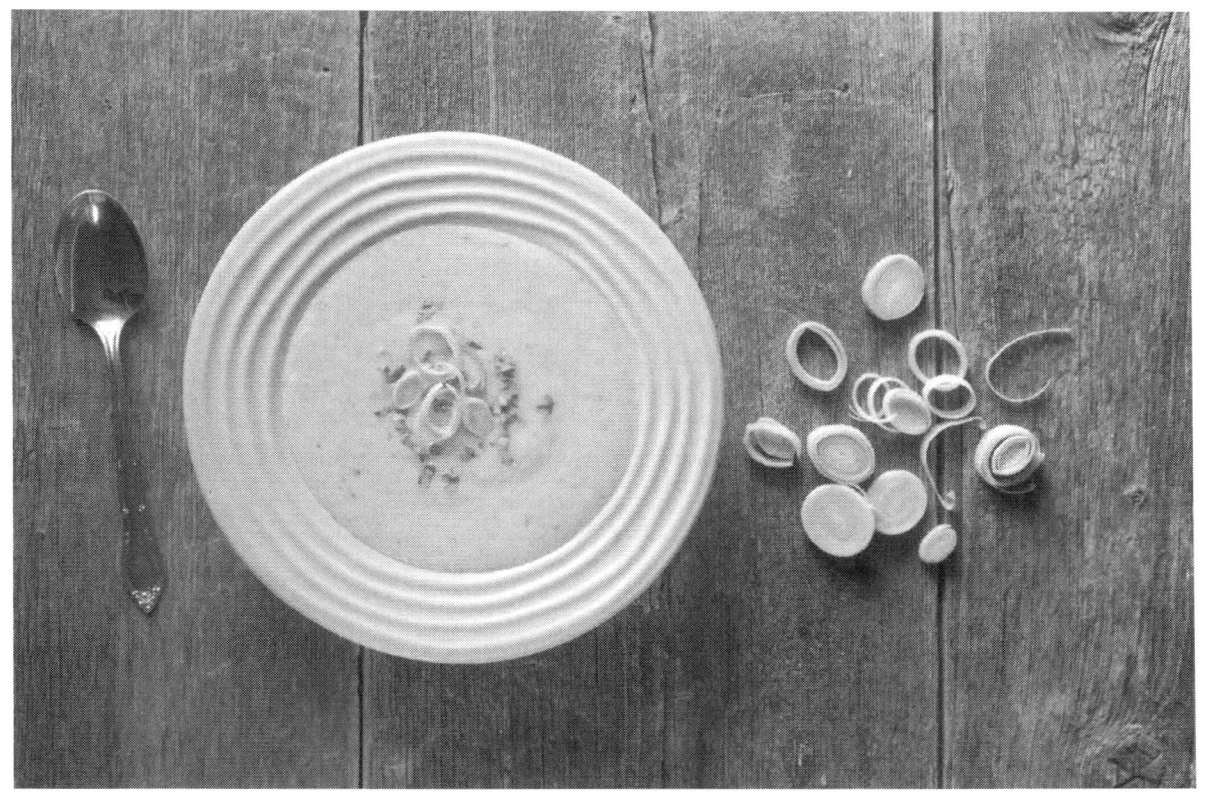

DELICIOUS LEEK CREAM SOUP

1 serving

Ingredients:

75ml of milk (low fat)

70g leek (cut into strips)

10g butter

1 teaspoon of cornflour

15g of processed cheese

A bit of paprika powder

25g of cream

125ml vegetable brew

Chives

Salt, pepper, nutmeg

Soups

Preparation:

Put the leek in the steami application of the cooking machine. Then pour the broth into the mix pot. Now insert the steam application with the leek and cook for 15 minutes at stage 1. When it is done use the spatula to remove the application. Add the starch and stir for 5 seconds at level 5.

Now add half of the leek and put the rest of it into a bowl. Now add butter, cream, milk and spices and cook for 6 minutes at stage 1 (100 degrees). Two minutes before it is done add the processed cheese. Season according to taste. Then put it to the remaining leek into the bowl. Ready to serve.

Nutritional values per 100ml:

KCAL	PRO	CAR	FAT
270	7g	14g	19g

LOW CARB CAULIFLOWER SOUP

1 serving

Ingredients:

1 ½ teaspoon oil

¼ garlic clove (small)

1 small piece of cauliflower

¼ onion

250ml vegetable stock

1 small carrot

15g cheese

1 teaspoon of cream

Preparation:

Peel the garlic and the onions and chop them at stage 5 for 8 seconds. Slide it down with the spatula and then steam at stage 1 (100 degrees) for 3 minutes. Chop the cauliflower coarsely and peel the carrots, cut them into pieces. Then add them to the mix pot as well as cheese and cream. Puree from stage 4 to 8 for 1 minute each stage. Serve in a bowl.

Nutritional values per 100ml:

KCAL	PRO	CAR	FAT
188	11g	13g	9g

Main dishes

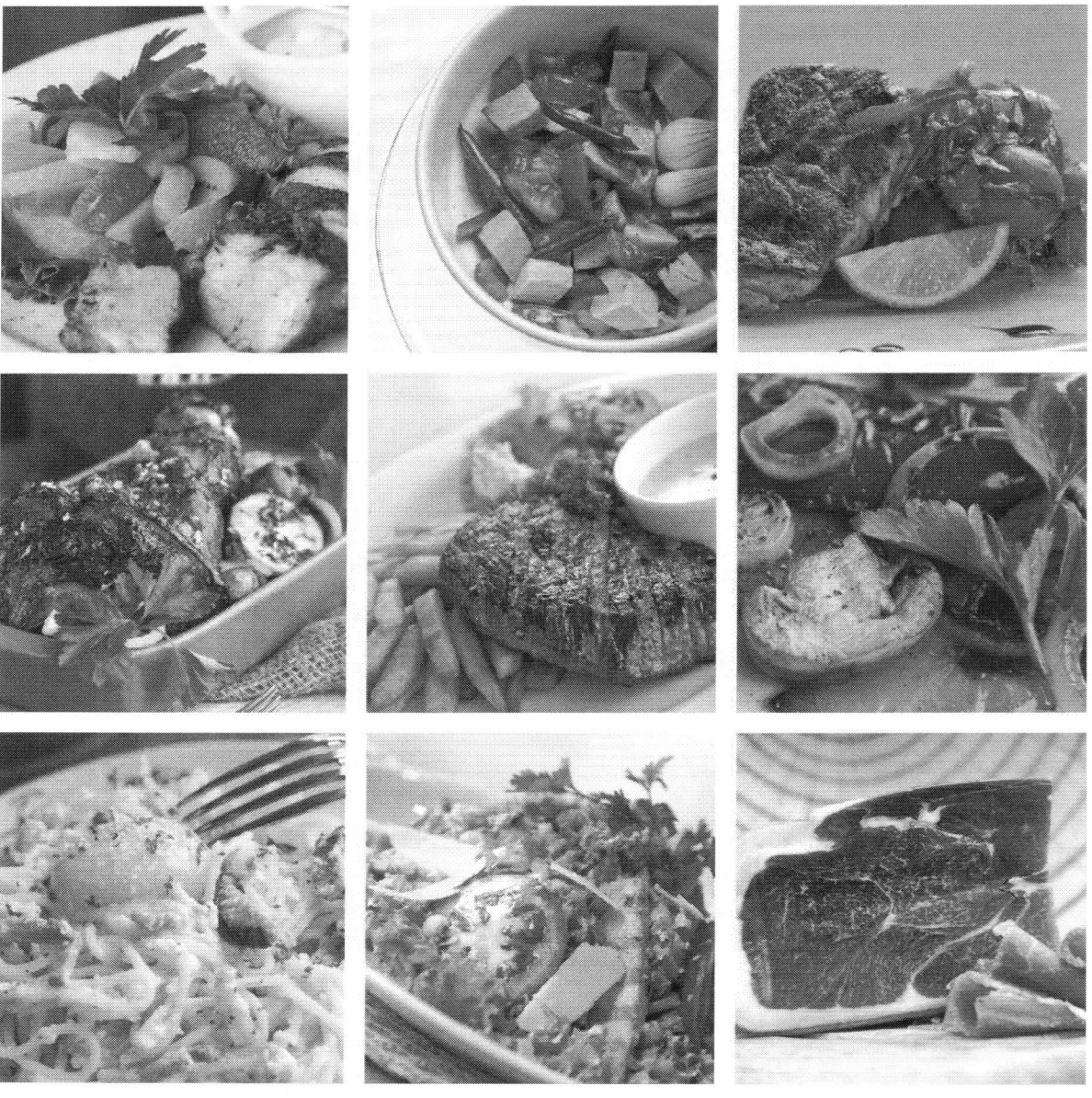

MAIN DISHES

Egg salad with shrimps 46

Spicy chicken breast salad 48

Superfood salad 50

Sausage salad with white cabbage 51

Italian salad bowl 53

Chicken fillet with tomatoes 54

Gratinated chicken pan 56

Shredded Pork with chili 58

Beef with chanterelles 59

Vegetable pan with salmon fillet 61

Cod in mustard sauce 62

Goulash 64

Low Carb chicken curry 65

Tuna-ricotta tortilla 67

Homemade pizza 78

Main dishes

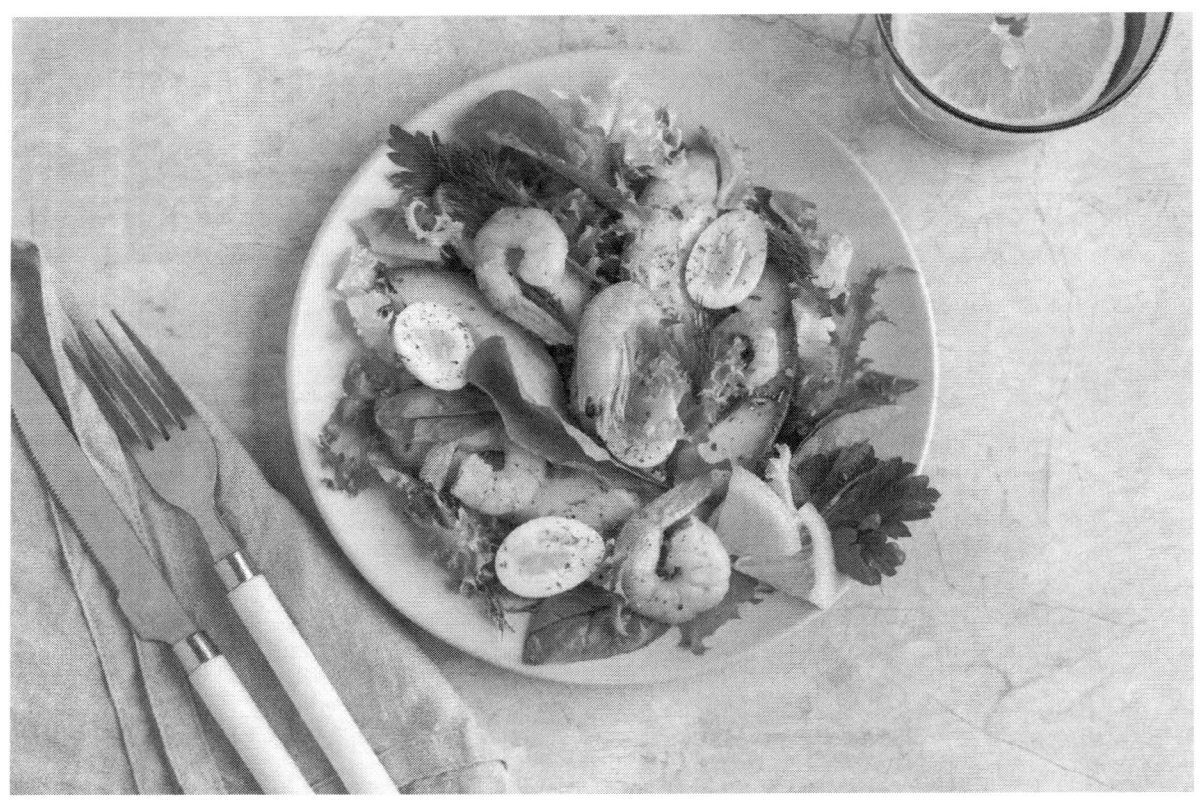

EGG SALAD WITH SHRIMPS

2 servings

Ingredients:

2 eggs

4 teaspoons of mayonnaise

6 teaspoons of yogurt

100g of romaine lettuce

1 clove of garlic

Half a pack of shrimps (ready to cook)

Salt, pepper, sweetener

½ bunch of chives

Preparation:

Boil the eggs for about 9 minutes. Then plunge into a pot of cold water. Then rinse with cold water and pee theml. Wash the chives and cut it into small rolls. Add the mayonnaise and yogurt to the mix pot. Then add pepper, salt and sweetener and shred coarsely at stage 8 for 5 seconds. Now add chives, eggs and shrimps to the mix pot and mix it at stage 1 in left running mode for 5 seconds. Season according to taste. Wash the lettuce and tear it into bite-sized pieces. The salat is ready to serve.

KCAL	PRO	CAR	FAT
300	9g	6g	26g

Main dishes

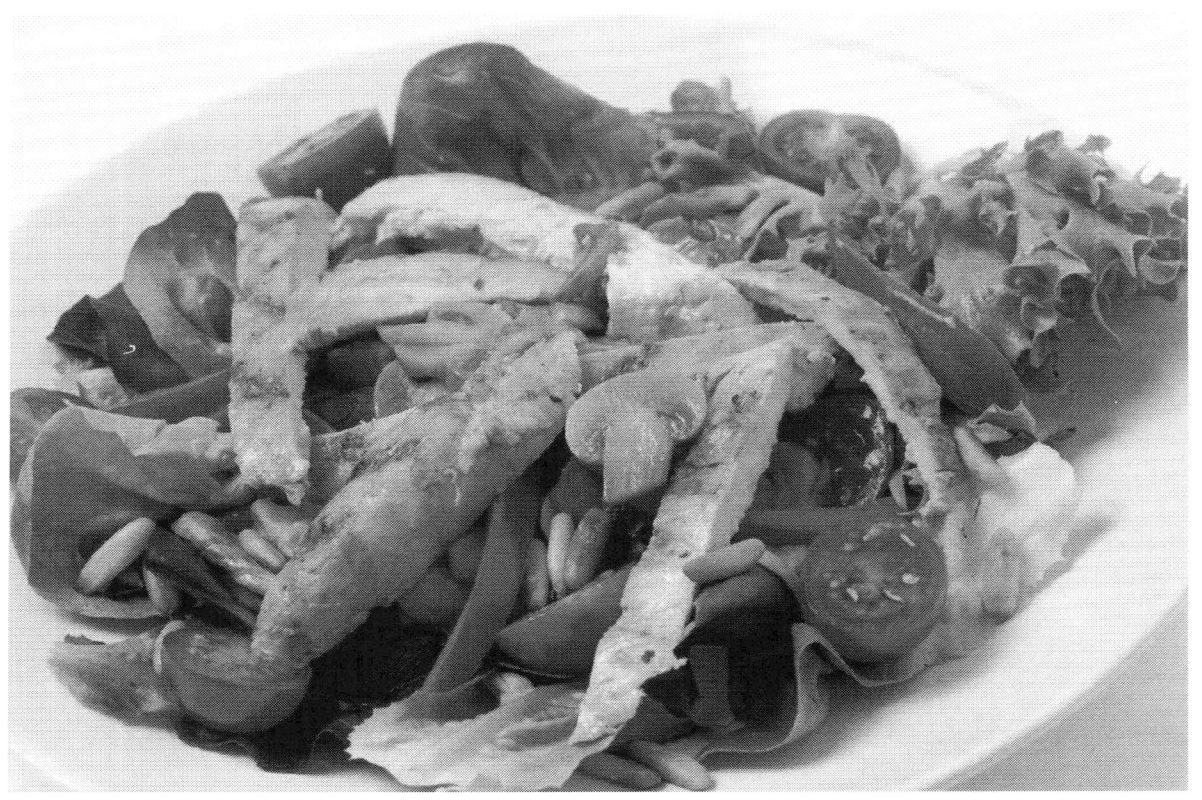

SPICY CHICKEN BREAST SALAD

2 servings

Ingredients:

200g chicken breast

25g of parmesan cheese

1 chilli pepper

1 teaspoon of soy sauce

½ red onion

100g cherry tomatoes

50g of arugula

100g of romaine lettuce

Main dishes

50g radicchio salad

2 teaspoons of balsamic vinegar

3 teaspoons of olive oil

Salt, pepper, chili powder, cayenne pepper

2 stalks of basil

1 stalk of parsley

Preparation:

Wash the chicken breast and pat dry. Cut it into coarsely pieces. Then cut the chili peppers and put them in a bowl. Add soy sauce, cayenne pepper and chili powder. Then add the chicken breast stripes and let it marinate.

Put the Parmesan cheese into the mix pot and shred it at stage 8 for 5 seconds. Then take it out of the mix pot and put it into a separate bowl. Take the meat out of the marinade and put it into the cooking machine. Add 1 teaspoon of oil and heat at at stage 2 (100 degrees) on left running mode for 6 minutes.

Wash the herbs, dry and pluck off the leaves. Add herbs, salt, pepper, vinegar and the remaining oil to the mix pot and mix at stage 8 for 4 seconds. Serve the ingredients on a plate.

KCAL	PRO	CAR	FAT
320	30g	5g	17g

Main dishes

SUPERFOOD SALAD

2 servings

Ingredients:

250g of broccoli

125g mushrooms

200g carrots

1 avocado

½ pomegranate

Half a lime

3 teaspoons of olive oil

50g of linseed

Salt, pepper, sweetener

Half a bunch of coriander

Preparation:

Wash the broccoli and cut it into florets. Cut the stalks into thin slices. Then cook both the sliced stalks and the florets in salted water for 8 minutes. Drain and rinse with cold water. Quarter the pomegranates and remove the seeds. Wash the mushrooms and peel the carrots. Put it all into the mix pot and shred for 5 seconds at stage 7. Then decant it.

Halve the avocados and remove the stone. Peel out the pulp with a spoon and cut it into small cubes. Squeeze the lime and pour the lime juice into the mix pot. Add salt, sweetener, pepper and oil. Then wash the coriander and pluck off the leaves. Add half of the leaves to the mix pot and mix the ingredients at stage 8 for 4 seconds and then again mix at stage 2 on left running mode for 3 seconds. Add the pomegranate seeds and the broccoli florets and mix for 3 seconds. Then put it into a salad bowl and garnish with the remaining coriander leaves.

KCAL	PRO	CAR	FAT
520	13g	12g	47g

Main dishes

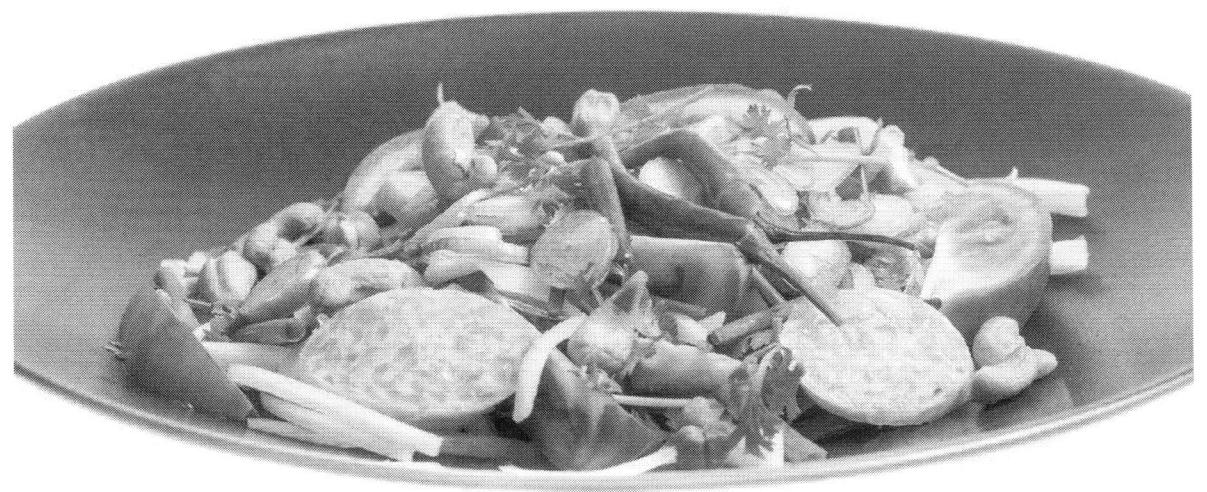

SAUSAGE SALAD WITH WHITE CABBAGE

2 servings

Ingredients:

20g walnuts

20g raisins

100g Meunster cheese

125g pork sausage

250g of white cabbage

1 teaspoon of sweet mustard

1 teaspoon of cider vinegar

1 teaspoon of walnut oil

Salt, pepper, sweetener

2 stalks of parsley

Main dishes

Preparation:

Brush the cabbage, then wash it and put it in the mix pot. Shred it at stage 7 for 10 seconds. Add mustard, sweetener, vinegar, pepper, oil and salt and mix at stage 3 in left running mode for 10 seconds. Then place it in the refrigerator and leave it for about 1 hour. Cut the sausage into thin slices. Then put the cheese into the mix pot and crush at stage 8 for 4 seconds. Then add the sausages, nuts and raisins as well as the cabbage. Season with salt and pepper and mix at stage 1 on left running mode for 10 seconds. Wash the parsley, dry well and pluck off the leaves. Arrange the salad in a bowl and sprinkle over the parsley.

KCAL	PRO	CAR	FAT
510	22g	14g	41g

Main dishes

ITALIAN SALAD BOWL

2 servings

Ingredients:

25g bresaola ham

65g buffalo mozzarella

50g of radicchio

1 red chili pepper

1 zucchini

1 clove of garlic

2 teaspoons olive oil

4 teaspoons balsamic vinegar

Salt pepper

2 sprigs of rosemary

1 stalk of basil

Preparation:

Wash the chili peppers, remove the cores and then cut them into fine stripes. Wash the zucchini, halve it and cut it into thin slices as well. Peel the garlic. Wash the rosemary and let it dry. Wash the basil and pluck off the leaves. Put 1 teaspoon of oil into the mix pot and then add the zucchini.

Now add the garlic and the rosemary and fry at stage 2 (100 degrees) in left running mode for 3 minutes. Add salt, pepper and 2 teaspoons of vinegar. Then decant it into a separate bowl. Now wash the arugula and tear it into bite-sized pieces. Cut the mozzarella into small cubes. Then put fried vegetables, arugula, mozzarella and the ham in a bowl and garnish with basil. Ready to serve!

KCAL	PRO	CAR	FAT
280	15g	5g	22g

Main dishes

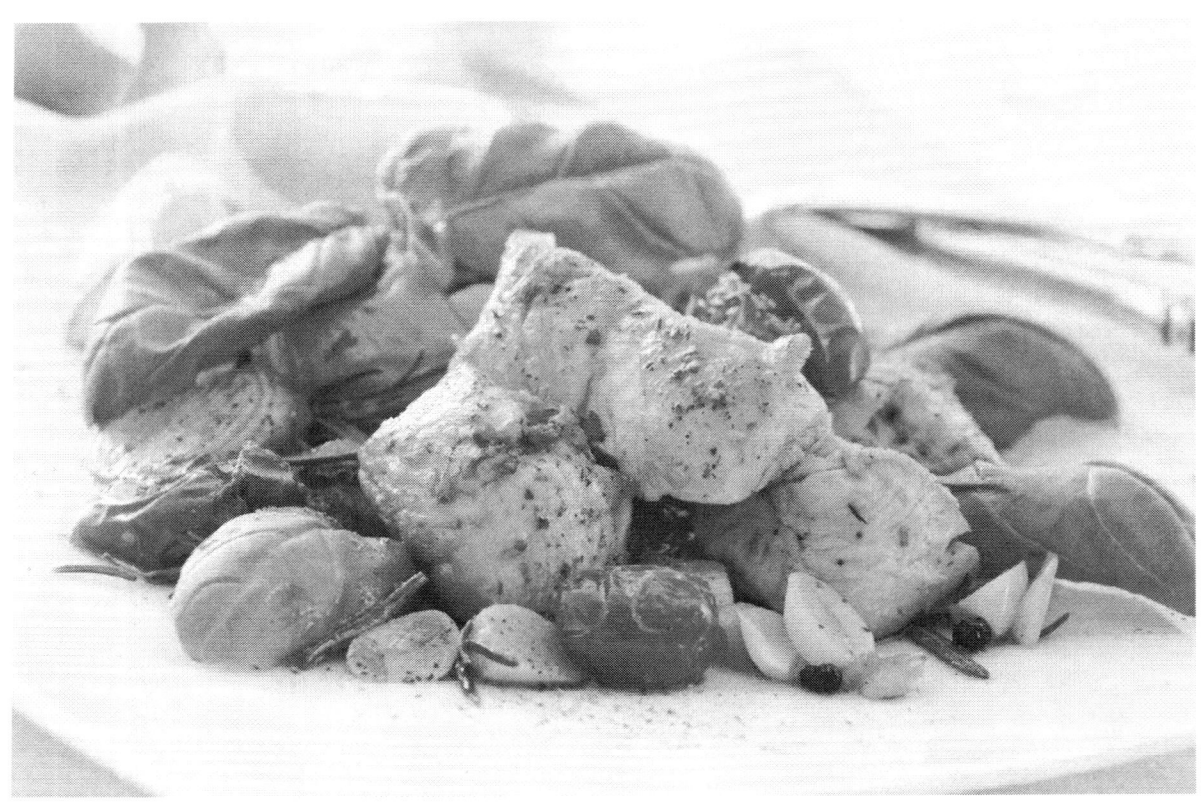

CHICKEN FILLET WITH TOMATOES

2 servings

Ingredients:

600g cherry tomatoes
250g chicken fillet
2 small red onions
2 cloves of garlic
1 red chilli
1 teaspoons of olive oil

Half a lemon
Salt, pepper
3 stalks of basil

Main dishes

Preparation:

Wash the tomatoes and the chicken fillet and let it dry thoroughly. Then cut the tomatoes into quarters. Peel the onions and the garlic and pour it into the mix pot. Now add the chilli peppers and chop at stage 5 for 4 seconds. Then decant it into a separate bowl. Cut the chicken fillet into stripes and put them into the mix pot. Now roast at stage 1 (100 degrees) in left running mode for 3 minutes.

Then add onions, garlic, tomatoes and chili peppers and fry for 5 minutes. Wash the lemon with hot water, peel off the lemon zest and squeeze out the juice. Wash the basil, dry and pluck off the leaves. Now put the lemon zest and the lemon juice as well as salt, pepper and half of the basil leaves into the mix pot and cook at stage 1 in left running mode for 1 minute. Season with spice and garnish with the remaining basil leaves.

KCAL	PRO	CAR	FAT
240	31g	12g	6g

Main dishes

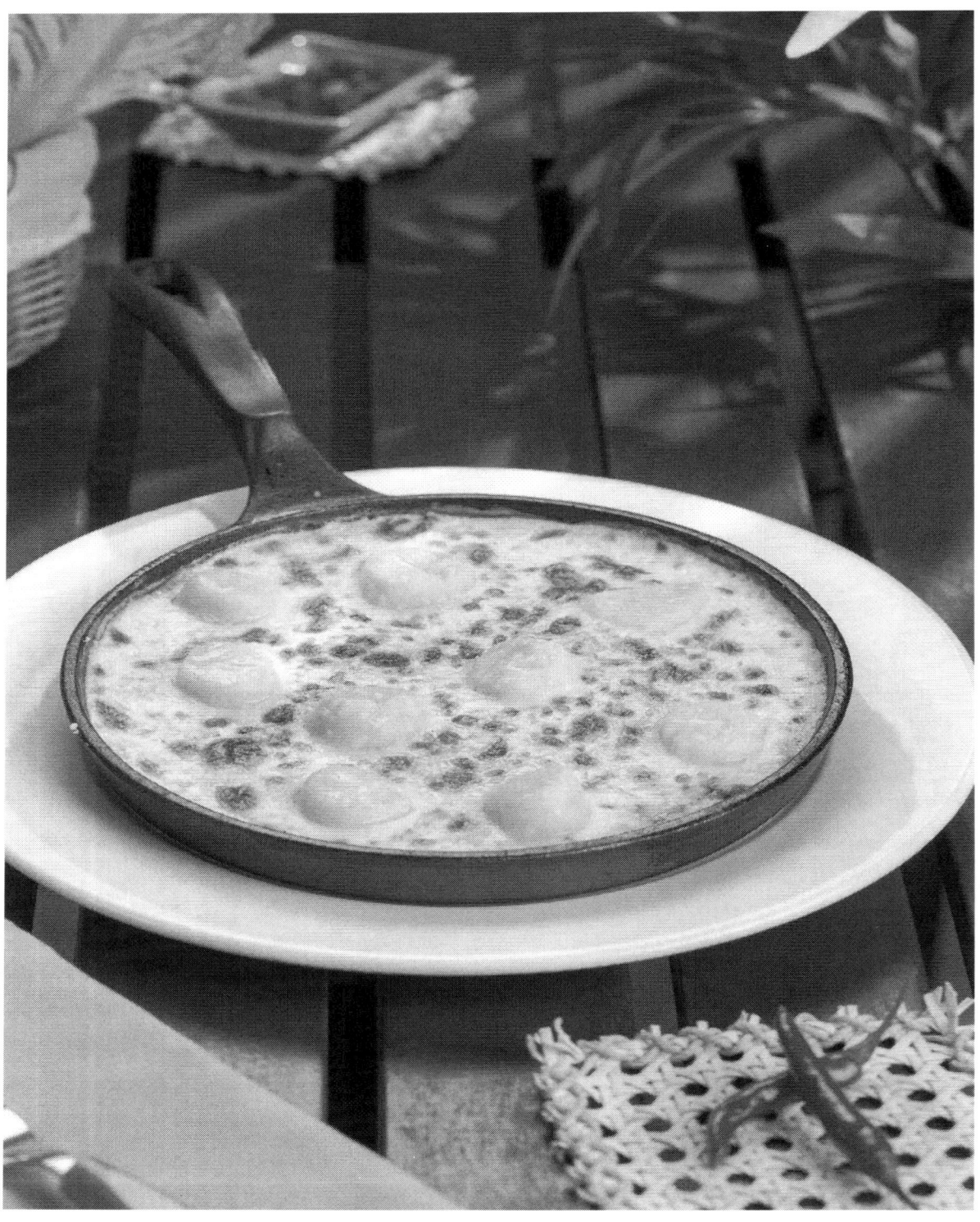

Main dishes

GRATINATED CHICKEN PAN

2 Servings

Ingredients:

200g chicken fillet

250g Brussels sprouts

250g broccoli

1 onion

75g chanterelles

50g cheese

30g fat

1 teaspoon of breadcrumbs (e.g. almond flour)

Salt, pepper

3 stalks parsley

Preparation:

Brush brussels sprouts and broccoli. Then cut the broccoli into florets. Wash the chicken and peel the onion. Then wash and clean the chanterelles thoroughly. Put the brussels sprouts and the broccoli into the Varoma application. Now pour in salted water and replace the Varoma. Add the chicken and close the Varoma application. Cook for 15 minutes at stage 1. Remove the Varoma application and put the vegetables on a sieve.

Place the chicken on a baking sheet. Put the bacon and the onion into the mix pot and shred at stage 5 for 4 seconds. Add oil and fry at stage 1 (100 degrees) on left running mode for 1 minute. Add chanterelles and fry for another 30 seconds. Then add the brussels sprouts and the broccoli and steam for 20 seconds. Decant it to the chicken in an ovenproof bowl.

Rinse the mix pot. Put the cheese in and chop at stage 5 for 3 seconds. Add the breadcrumbs and mix at stage 2 for 4 seconds. Now sprinkle the mixture over the chicken and bake in preheated oven at 225 degrees for 10 minutes. When the cheese is melted, wash the parsley, dry well and pluck off the leaves. Garnish the chicken with it.

KCAL	PRO	CAR	FAT
540	41g	12g	37g

Main dishes

SHREDDED PORK WITH CHILI

2 servings

Ingredients:

300g minute steaks from pork

1 red onion

1 clove of garlic

2 red peppers

2 teaspoons olive oil

50ml vegetable stock

2 tablespoons creme fraiche

2 teaspoons pine nuts

1 teaspoon Parmesan

Salt pepper

5 stalks basil

Preparation:

Wash the basil well and put it in the mix pot. Add the pine nuts, 1 teaspoon of olive oil, Parmesan cheese and salt and shred at level 10 for 4 seconds to a pesto. Then decant. Cut the meat into thin stripes and peel onion and garlic. Wash, halve and remove the seeds from the chili peppers. Now put the vegetables into the mix pot and shred at stage 7 for 5 seconds. Then decant it into a separate bowl.

Now put the remaining oil into the mix pot, add the meat and fry at stage 2 (100 degrees) in left running mode for 5 minutes. Add the vegetables and fry with the meat for 30 seconds. Then deglaze with vegetable brew and simmer at stage 1 in left running mode for 8 minutes. Season with salt and pepper. Add creme fraiche and the pesto and mix at stage 2 for 5 seconds in left running mode. Season to taste. Ready to serve.

KCAL	PRO	CAR	FAT
240	25g	8g	12g

Main dishes

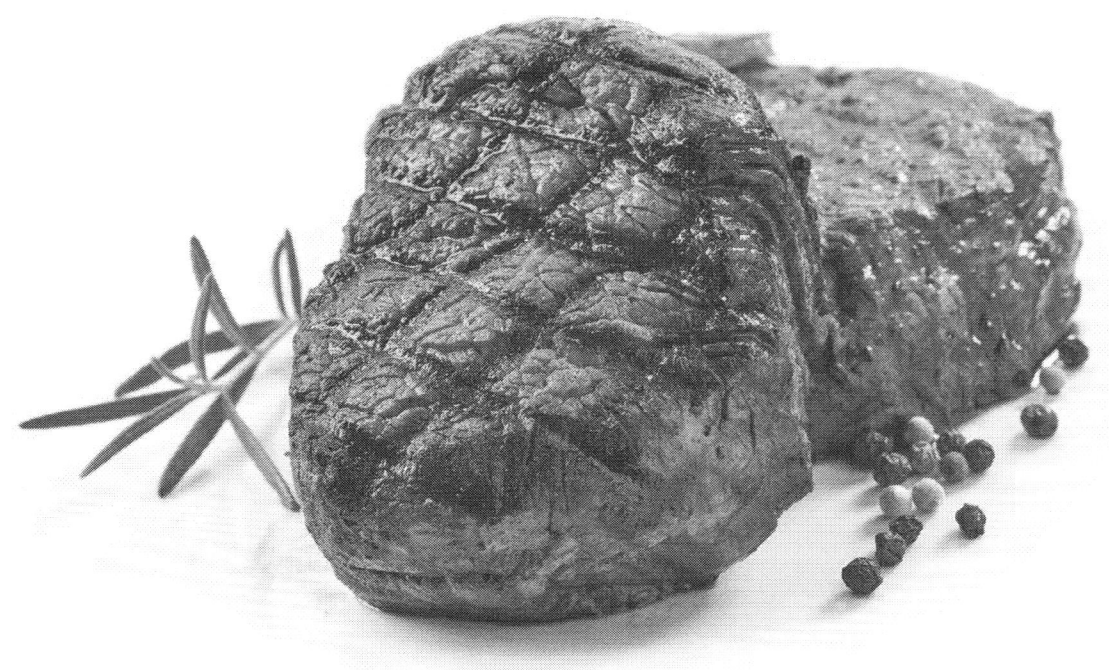

BEEF WITH CHANTERELLES

2 servings

Ingredients:

125g beef

100g chanterelles

2 shallots

35g fat

2 teaspoons canola oil

½ lemon

1 clove of garlic

3 tsp Balsamic Vinegar

Salt pepper

2 stalks parsley

1 stalk thyme

Main dishes

Preparation:

Brush the chanterelles and wash them. Peel the shallots and the garlic. Wash the herbs and pluck off the leaves. Cut the beef into thin slices and then add the shallots and the garlic to the mix pot. Crush at stage 5 for 4 seconds. Then decant. Then put the bacon into the mix pot and shred at stage 5 for 3 seconds. Then fry at 100 degrees at stage 1 for 2 minutes. Add 1 teaspoon of canola oil and the chanterelles and fry at stage 1 for 2 minutes.

Then add shallots, herbs and the garlic and cook for another 20 seconds. Season with salt and pepper. Add the vinegar and then simmer for 10 seconds. Now decant into a bowl and let it cool. Put the remaining oil into the mix saucepan, add the beef and cook at stage 1 (120 degrees) in left running mode for 20 seconds. Serve on a plate and season with salt and pepper.

KCAL	PRO	CAR	FAT
310	16g	2g	25g

VEGETABLE PAN WITH SALMON FILLET

2 servings

Ingredients:

300g salmon fillet

1 red onion

1 zucchini

1 yellow carrot

1 fennel bulb

3 tsp sunflower oil

½ lemon

50g cream cheese

1 tsp vegetable stock, instant

Salt pepper

2 stalks dill

2 stalks lemon thyme

Preparation:

Peel the onion as well as the zucchini and the carrots. Brush the fennel and wash it. Cut the green of the fennel off. Give the chopped vegetables into the mix pot and chop at stage 5 for 8 seconds. Now put the vegetables in the Varoma application and cover the inlaid floor of the Varoma with parchment paper. Place the salmon on it. Then pour the salt water into the mix pot. Now insert the Varoma application and the inlaid floor and close it. Steam at stage 1 for 15 minutes. Wash the herbs, then dry them and pluck off the leaves and needles.

Then add oil and vegetables and fry at stage 2 (120 °C) in left running mode for 1 minute. Squeeze out a lemon and add the juice. Season with salt and pepper. Continue frying for another 20 seconds. Then add 150 ml of water, cream cheese and instant broth. Cook at stage 1 in left running mode for 2 minutes. Serve it with the salmon and sprinkle with herbs.

KCAL	PRO	CAR	FAT
497	35g	8g	34g

Main dishes

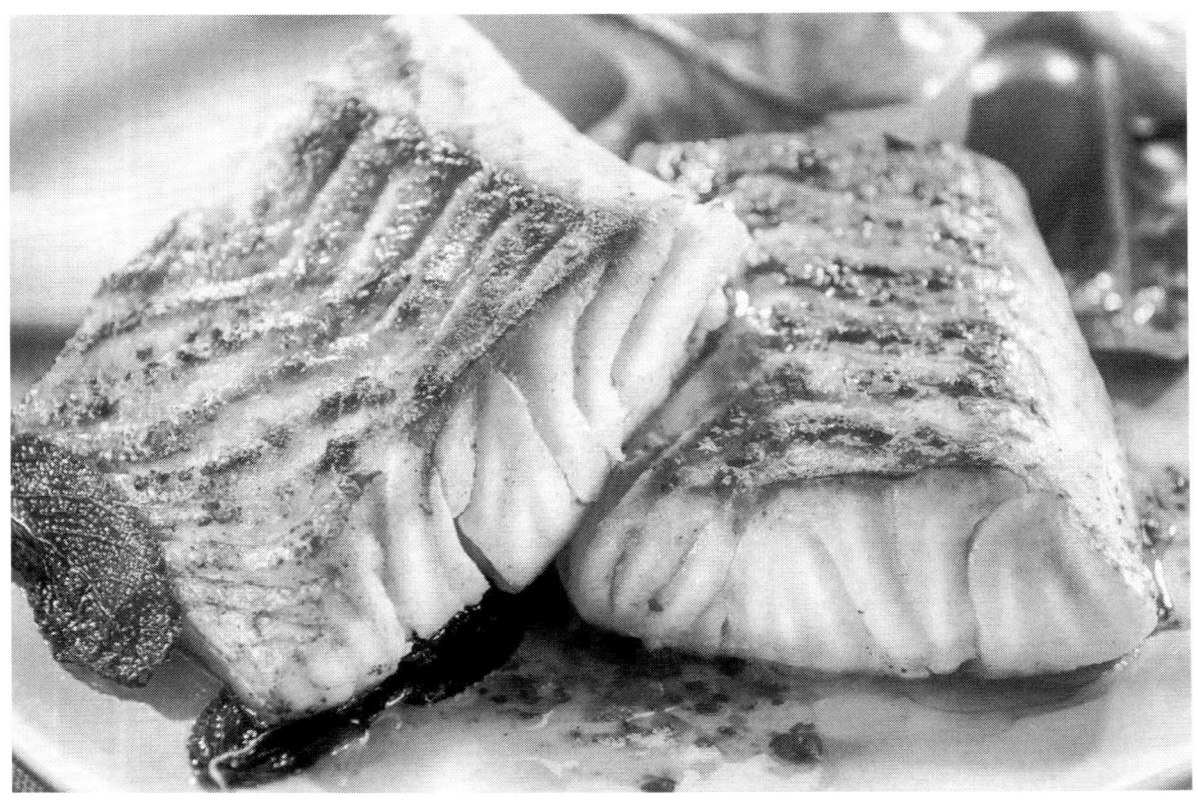

COD IN MUSTARD SAUCE

1 serving

Ingredients:

150g cod fillet

2 ½ teaspoons of white wine

1 egg yolk

½ teaspoon of oil

1 teaspoon of tarragon mustard

½ teaspoon of whipped cream or soy cream

Salt, white pepper

Main dishes

Preparation:

Rinse the fish with cold water, then pat dry. Now spice it up well. Whip the yolk with mustard and white wine in the mix-pot for 5 minutes until it is creamy. Then pour the cream into it and stir. Season with salt and pepper. Decant the sauce and keep it warm. Cover the Varoma application with oil. Put the cod in Varoma application and steam for 8-10 minutes under high heat. Put it out after 5 minutes and serve it with sauce.

Nutritional values per 100g:

KCAL	PRO	CAR	FAT
261	30g	0g	13g

GOULASCH

1 serving

Ingredients:

175g goulash mixed

150ml beef stock

50g mushrooms, fresh

⅔ chili pepper, fresh

⅓ garlic

⅓ onion, red

¼ onion, diced

20g tomato puree

4 tablespoons of white wine

Clarified butter

Sweet paprika

Hot pepper

Salt, pepper, chili powder

Preparation:

Fry onions and garlic with butter in the cooking machine. Then add paprika, tomato paste, mushrooms, beef broth and white wine. Simmer the goulasch at 100 degrees for 45 minutes at stage 1. If necessary, reduce fluid to thicken the goulasch. Then season with the spices.

Nutritional values per 100g:

KCAL	PRO	CAR	FAT
47	4g	1g	2g

Main dishes

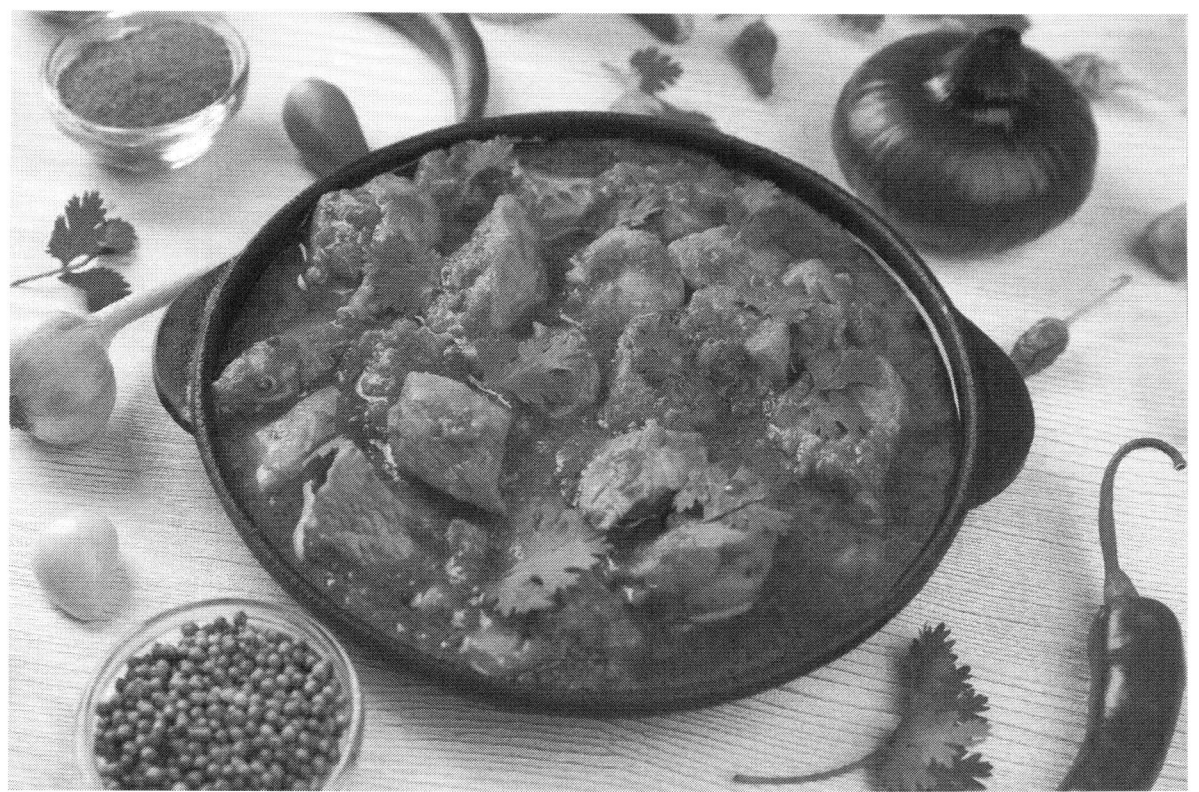

LOW CARB CHICKEN CURRY

1 serving

Ingredients:

175g of chicken breast

1 carrot or zucchini

3 teaspoons of soy sauce

1 cup of water

3 teaspoons of tomato paste

1 teaspoon of curry powder

1 pinch of sambal oelek

Salt, garlic

Main dishes

Preparation:

Wash the chicken breast, pat dry and cut it into small stripes. Mix the soy sauce with the Sambal Oelek and then marinate the chopped chicken breast at least 10 minutes in it. Wash the vegetables and cut them coarsely. Put the chicken breast and the marinade in the mix pot and steam at stage 3 (100° C). Enter the vegetables and steam again for another 3 minutes. Add tomato paste, curry powder and water. Cook while the stirring process continues until the vegetables are cooked al dente.

KCAL	PRO	CAR	FAT
340	43g	13g	11g

Main dishes

TUNA-RICOTTA TORTILLA

2 servings

Ingredients:

70g tuna fillet

1 teaspoon of pine nuts

1 clove of garlic

15g olives (without stone)

15g dried tomatoes in oil

10g of Parmesan cheese

2 teaspoons of breadcrumbs

2 eggs

120g of ricotta cheese

Salt, pepper

1 stalk of oregano

1 stalk of thyme

Preparation:

Put the Parmesan cheese and the breadcrumbs into the mix pot and crush at stage 8 for 4 seconds. Then decant it into a separate bowl. Peel the garlic, wash the herbs, dry well and pluck off the leaves. Now put the pine nuts into the mix pot and roast them without adding fat at 100 degrees at stage 1 fry for 3 minutes. Then decant them into a separate bowl. Put tomatoes, olives and garlic in the mix pot and shred everything at stage 5 for 3 seconds. Then decant into a separate vessel.

Separate the eggs and put the egg yolks with the ricotta into the mix pot. Add half of the Parmesan cheese. Then stir until the mixture is smooth and add salt with pepper and continue stirring at stage 3 for 3 seconds. Decant it. Clean the mix pot and add the egg whites. Whip them at stage 8 for 10 seconds until it is stiff. Mix gently with olives, garlic, tomatoes, tuna, herbs, pine nuts and egg yolk at stage 1 until it is mixed properly. Line the Varoma insert with baking paper and sprout over the remaining Parmesan cheese. Pour in the mixture. Pour 300 ml of water into the mix pot. Add the Varoma application and steam for 25 minutes at stage 1. Take the Ricotta carefully from the Varoma insert.

KCAL	PRO	CAR	FAT
260	16g	8g	18g

Main dishes

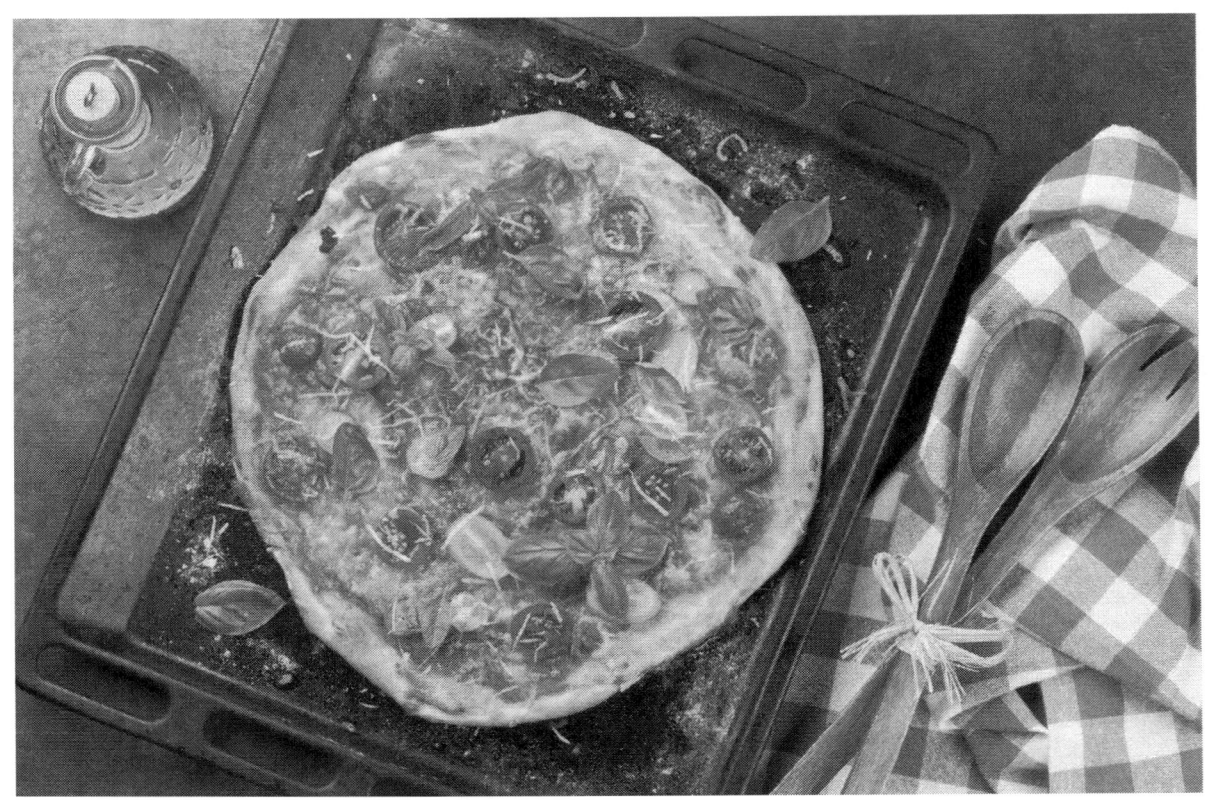

HOMEMADE PIZZA

1 serving

Ingredients:

35g cream cheese, low-fat

35g freshly grated Parmesan,

50ml tomato sauce

185g mozzarella

1 egg

3 teaspoons of low-fat whipped cream

⅓ garlic

Main dishes

Preparation:

Cover a baking sheet with oil and preheat oven to 180 degrees. Cut the mozzarella into thin slices and place the pieces of cheese on the sheet. Break the Parmesan and put it in the mixer. Then grind it finely at stage 10. Add the eggs, cream cheese, cream and garlic and mix for 10 seconds at stage 4.

Pour the egg-cheese mass over the mozzarella and bake it for 30 minutes on the lowest level in the oven. Take the mozzarella from the oven, cover with the pizza sauce and the desired ingredients. The pizza now takes another 10 to 15 minutes till it is done.

Nutritional values per 100g:

KCAL	PRO	CAR	FAT
217	16g	1g	16g

Vegetarian main dishes

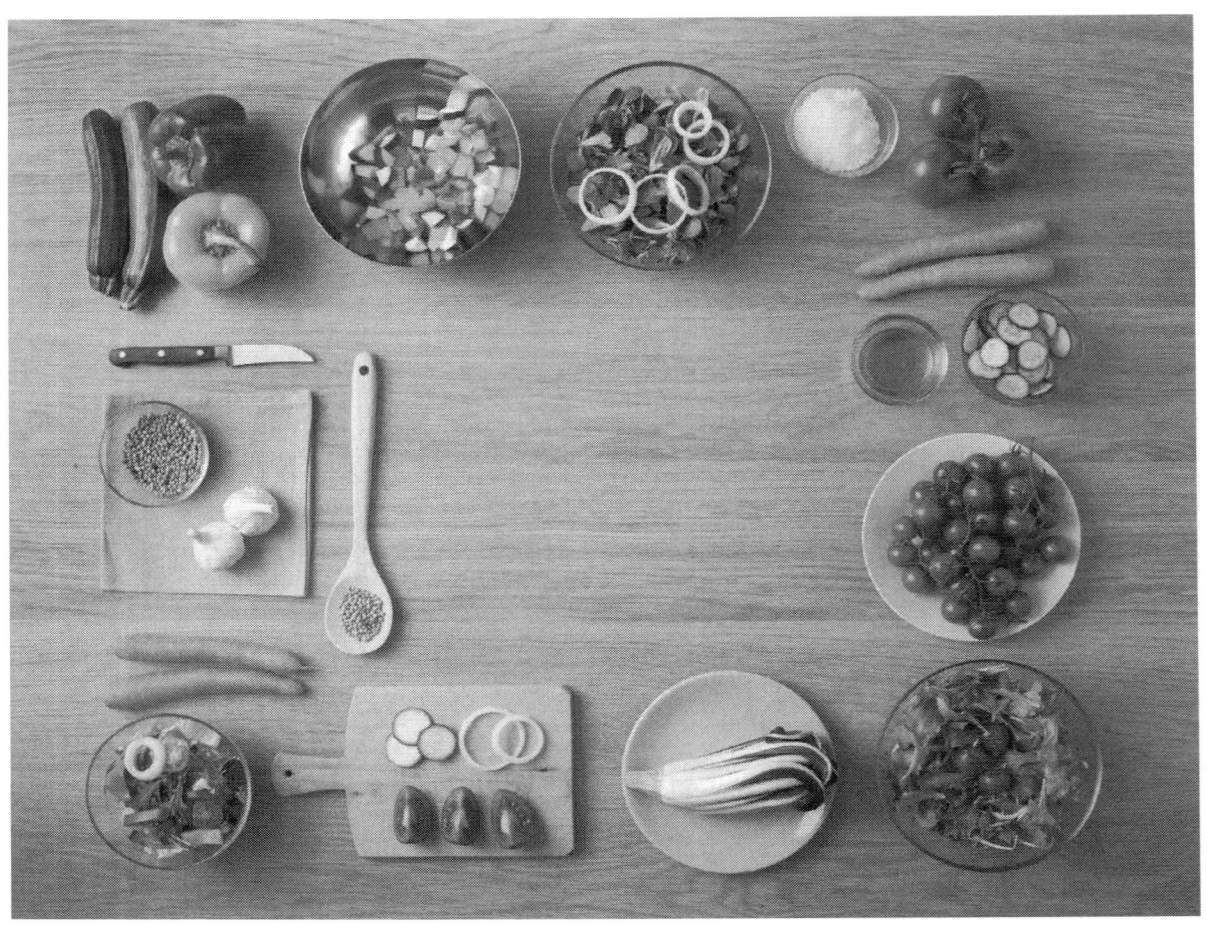

VEGETARIAN MAIN DISHES

Vegetable pasta with spinach and feta 71

Vegetable cheese pasta 73

Spicy carrot rosti 74

Leek pie 75

Ricotta Aubergine Gratin 76

Vegetarian main dishes

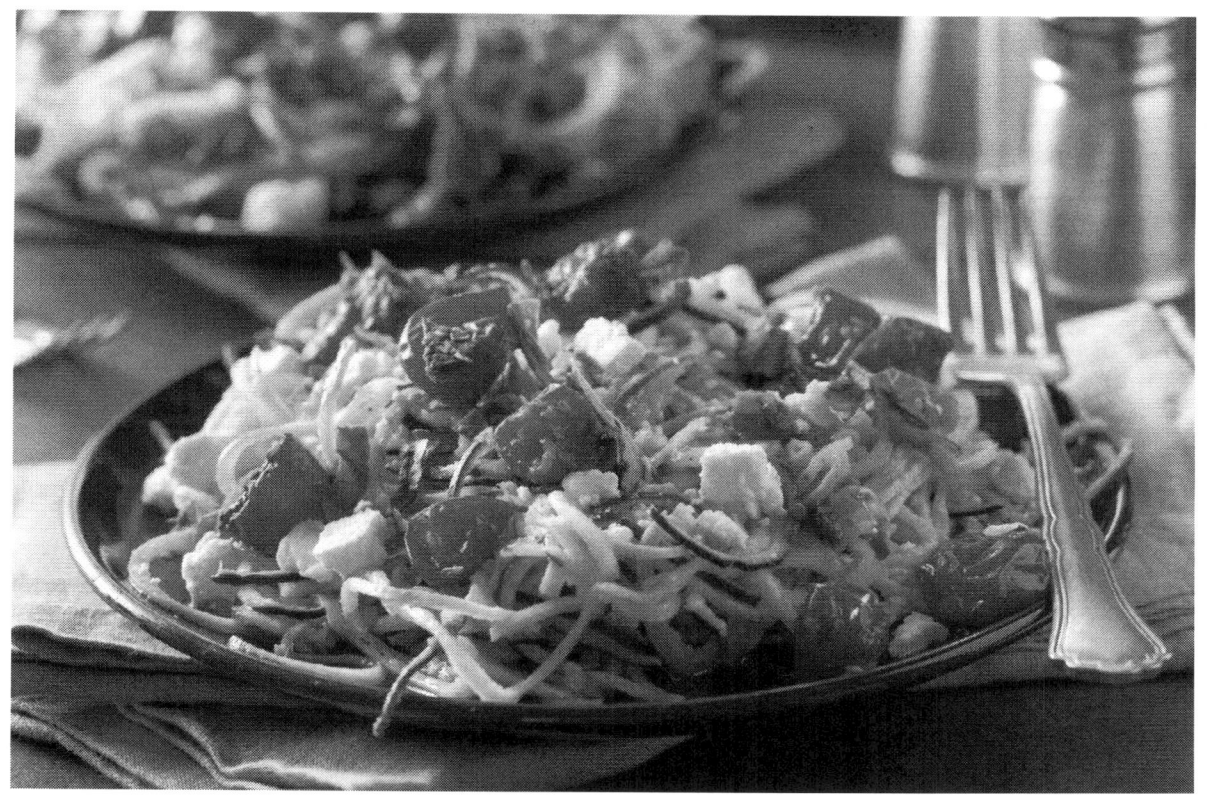

VEGETABLE PASTA WITH SPINACH AND FETA

1 serving

Ingredients:

65g spinach, fresh

25g feta cheese

1 ½ EL rapeseed oil

1 clove of garlic, to taste

320g courgettes

Salt

Vegetarian main dishes

Preparation:

Cut the zucchini with a spiral cutter in spirals. Steam the garlic for 8 seconds on stage 8. Slide it down with the spatula. Add the feta cheese and the spinach and shred and for 5 seconds at stage 8. Add salt and oil to the mix pot and stir for 10 seconds stage 5. Decant the spinach and cheese mixture and wash the mix pot.

Add 500ml of water to the mix pot and fry the vegetable noodles using the Varoma application for 12 minutes at stage 1. Then Put the zucchini noodles on a plate, spread the pesto over the pasta and garnish with feta.

KCAL	PRO	CAR	FAT
286	12g	9g	22g

Vegetarian main dishes

VEGETABLE CHEESE PASTA

1 serving

Ingredients:

125g carrots, peeled

125g courgette

70g mushrooms

1 spring onion

30g dried tomatoes

½ ball mozzarella

2 teaspoons olive oil

½ tsp salt

500ml water

Preparation:

Cut the zucchini and the carrots in spirals. Put the carrots spaghetti and the zucchini spaghetti in the Varoma application and cook for 12 minutes at stage 1. Now decant and put it aside. Then shred the mozzarella for 5 seconds at stage 4. Fill it in a bowl and rinse the mix pot.

Put mushrooms, spring onions, dried tomatoes and 1 teaspoon of olive oil into the mix pot and chop for 5 seconds at stage 4. Slide it down with the spatula and steam for 5 minutes at stage 1 (100°C). Now put the carrots and the zucchini with olive oil and salt in the mix saucepan and cook at stage 5 for 5 minutes. Arrange on plates and garnish with mozzarella.

KCAL	PRO	CAR	FAT
609	29g	11g	47g

Vegetarian main dishes

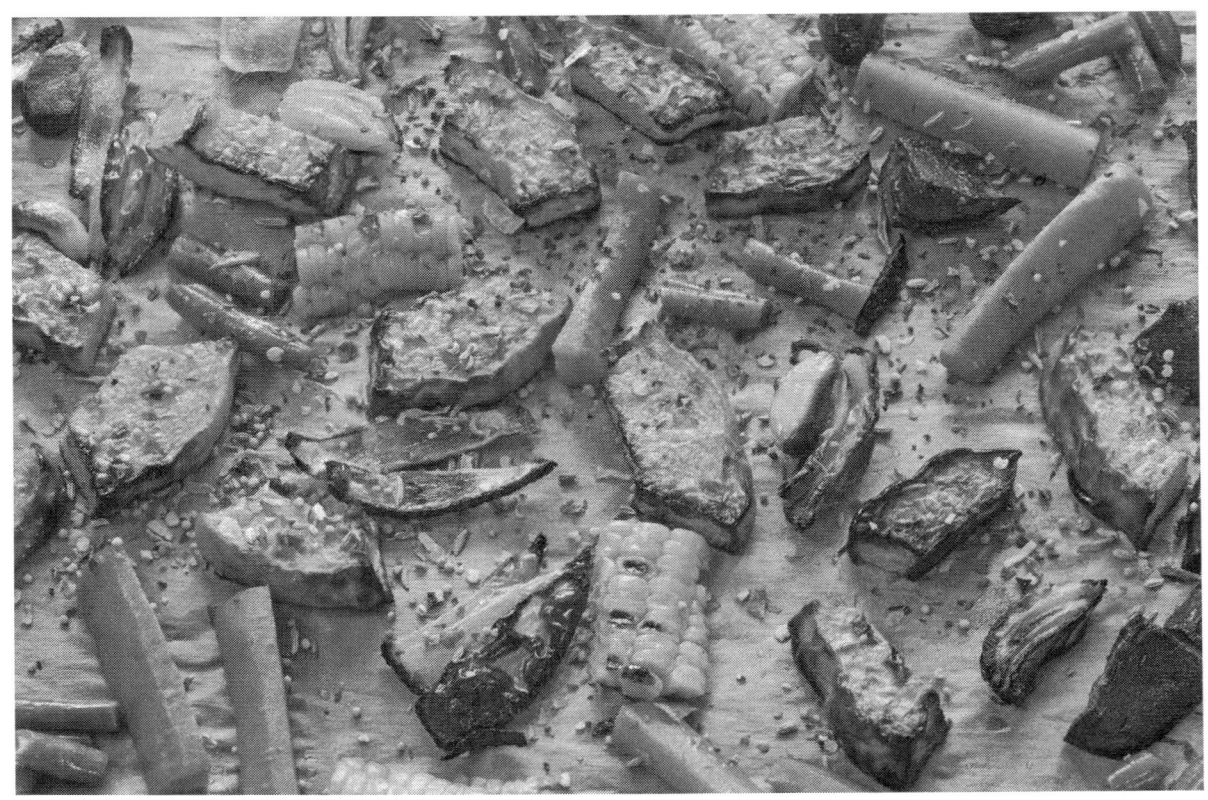

SPICY CARROT ROSTI

1 serving

Ingredients:

1 egg

1 piece of ginger, small

175g fresh carrots

pepper and salt

chilli flakes

Some oil

Preparation:
Wash the carrots and cut them into chunks. Peel the ginger, shred it at stage 10. Add the carrots and chop a few seconds at stage 4. Stir them and the eggs at stage 4 for 10 seconds. Season it with salt and pepper and sprinkle the chilli flakes over it. Heat oil in a pan and fry the rösti from both sides in it.

KCAL	PRO	CAR	FAT
239	9g	11g	16g

LEEK CAKE

1 serving

Ingredients:

2 eggs

220g of leek

180g of of sour cream

50g hard cheese

1 teaspoon of oil

Herbs, salt, pepper,

Garlic (according to taste)

Preparation:

Cut the cheese into small pieces and put it into the mix pot. Shred it at stage 8 for 10 seconds. Then decant it. Peel the porree and the garlic and chop it in the mix pot at stage 5 for 4 seconds. Push it down to the ground with the spatula down and stew with butter or oil with the Varoma application for 4 minutes at stage 1.

Add the eggs, cream cheese, salt, pepper, herbs and half of the grated cheese. Then stir it for 10 seconds at stage 3. Pour the mixture into a greased baking sheet. Sprinkle the remaining cheese over it, then bake the leek cake for 40 minutes at 180 degrees. Spice up with Oregano.

KCAL	PRO	CAR	FAT
673	34g	15g	50g

Vegetarian main dishes

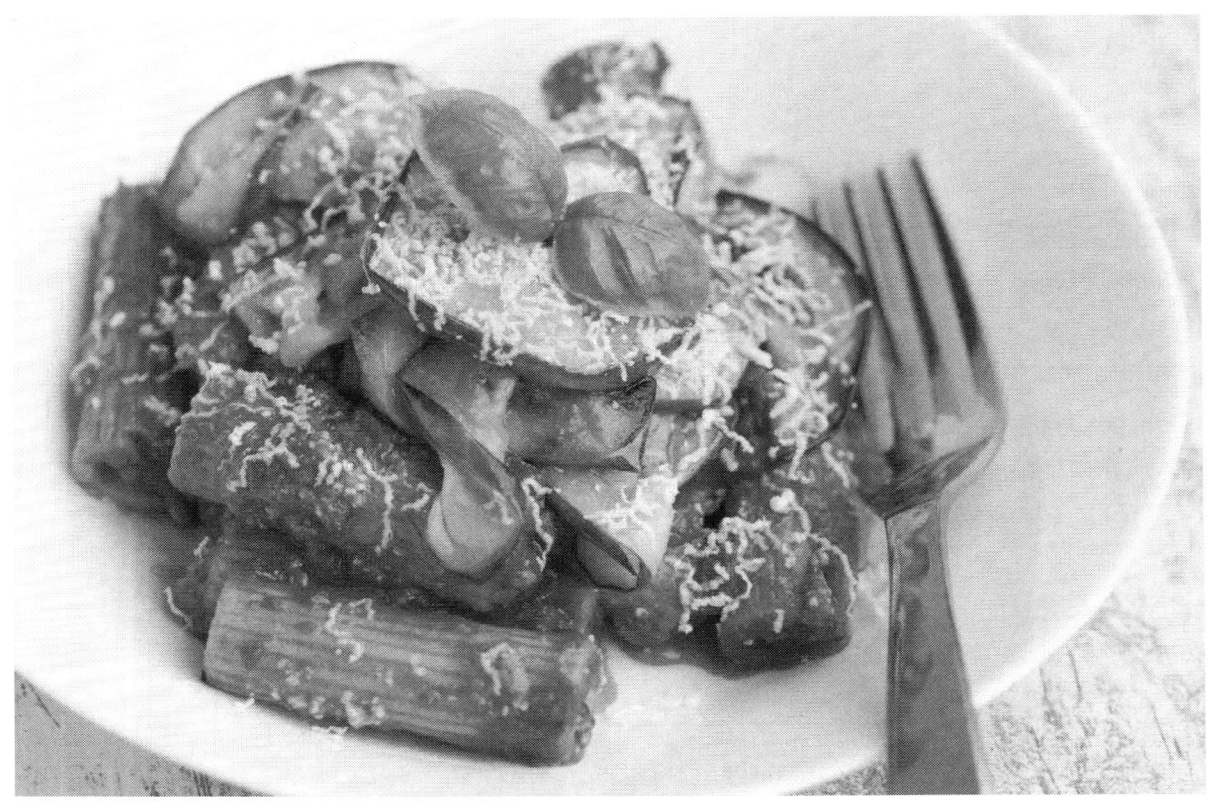

RICOTTA AUBERGINE GRATIN

2 servings

Ingredients:

600g aubergines

200g ricotta

1 clove of garlic

400ml canned tomatoes

30g parmesan

100ml low-fat milk

1 teaspoon olive oil

Salt pepper

2 stalks Oregano

2 stalks basil

Preparation:

Wash, halve and slice the eggplants. Spread a baking sheet with parchment paper and place the eggplants on it. Preheat oven at 175°C and cook them for 5 minutes under convection. Wash, dry and pluck the leaves off the herbs and peel the garlic. Add the Parmesan into the mix pot and shred it at stage 5 for 3 seconds. Decant it into a separate bowl. Now put the Parmesan cheese into the mix pot, add the milk and stir at stage 5 for 3 seconds. Add the ricotta cheese and stir for another 3 seconds. Decant it as well.

Add the garlic to the mix pot and chop it for 3 seconds at stage 5. Then add the tomatoes, as well as salt, pepper and herbs and mix on stage 5 for 4 seconds. Cover a baking sheet with oil and then stack the tomato sauce, the eggplants and the ricotta mousse each in layers on it. Sprinkle with Parmesan cheese and then bake the gratin in the oven for 30 minutes (with same temperature).

KCAL	PRO	CAR	FAT
400	27g	10g	24g

Smoothies

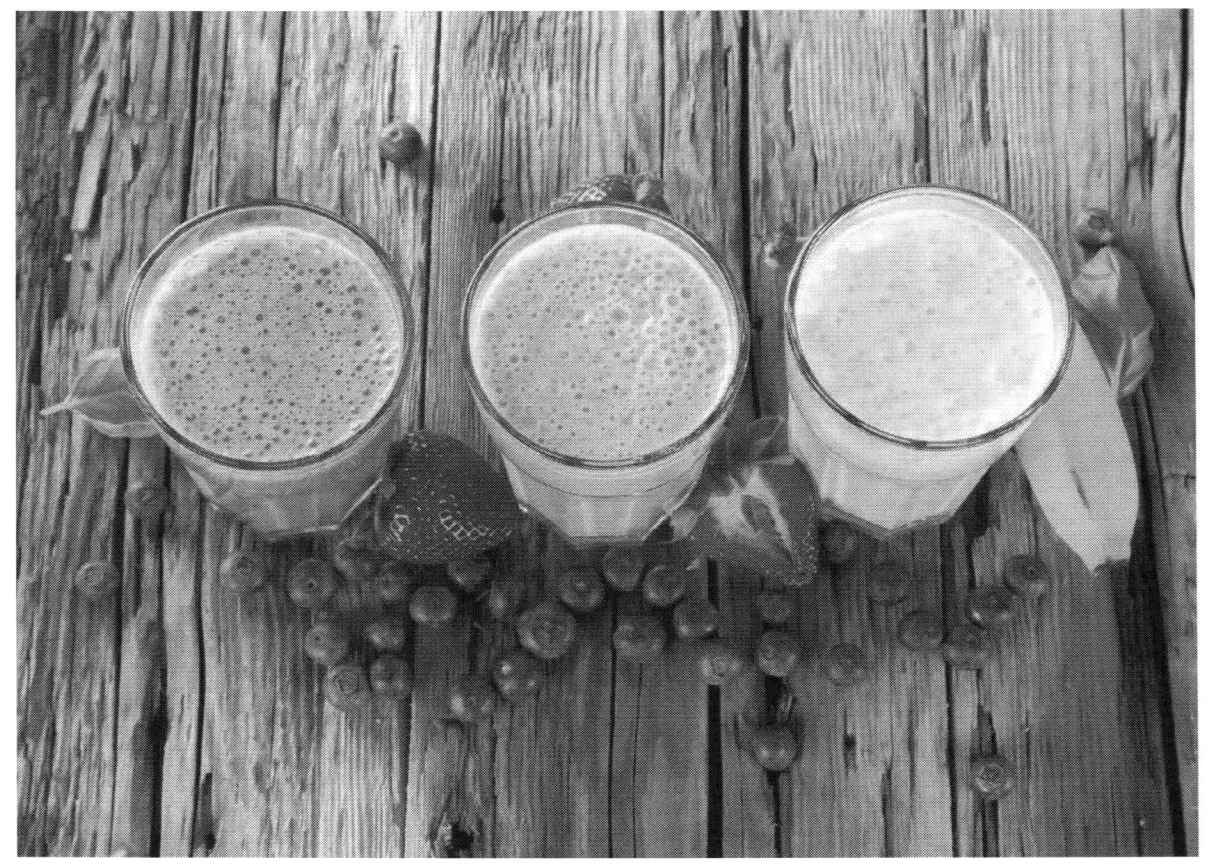

SMOOTHIES

Spring smoothie 80

Grapefruit and carrot smoothie 81

Spicy Ginger Curcuma smoothie..82

Fat Burner smoothie...84

Citrus and avocado smoothie...85

Smoothies

Cocos smoothie with carrots 86

Berry shake.. 87

Kiwi almond milk shake 88

Lettuce cucumber smoothie 89

Nectarine Orange smoothie 90

Smoothies

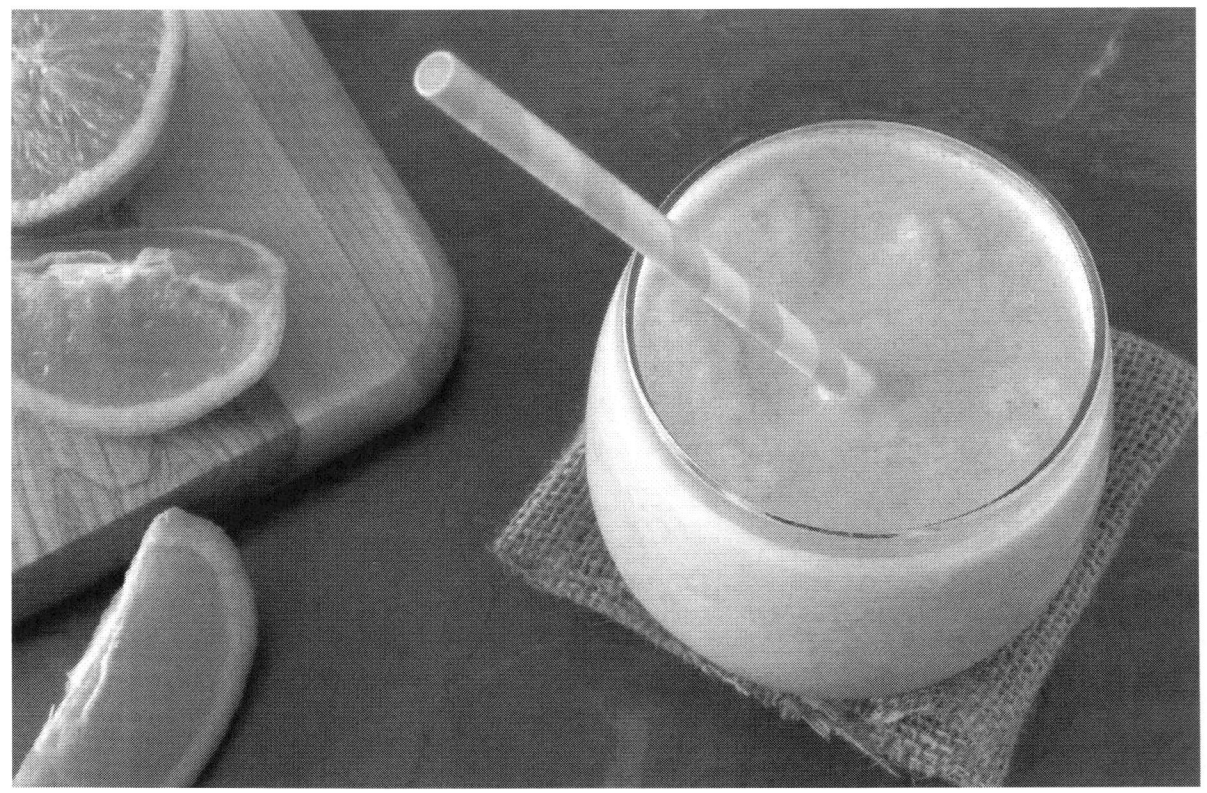

SPRING SMOOTHIE

2 servings

Ingredients:

20g lignite leaves
50g radish
1 kiwi
1 peach
1 lemon
100ml orange juice
150ml of water

Preparation:
Peel the kiwi, wash the peach, halve and core it. Wash the lemon with hot water, dry well and peel half of it to lemon zest. Squeeze out the lemon juice and put kiwi, peach, lemon peel, lemon juice, orange juice and water into the mixing pot and mix it for 10 seconds at stage 10 and serve fresh in two glasses.

KCAL	PRO	CAR	FAT
60	1g	10g	0g

GRAPEFRUIT CARROT SMOOTHIE

4 servings

Ingredients:

1kg carrots

5 pink grapefruits

2 stalks of mint

2 handful of ice cubes

Preparation:

Peel and clean the carrots. Halve the grapefruits and squeeze out the juice. Then wash the mint leaves. Halve the carrots and squeeze in the juicer to the carrot juice. Add the remaining carrots, the grapefruit juice, the freshly squeezed carrot juice, ice cubes and the mint leaves to the mixing pot and mix at stage 10 for 10 seconds. If the mass is too thick, just add some water.

KCAL	PRO	CAR	FAT
35	0g	6g	1g

Smoothies

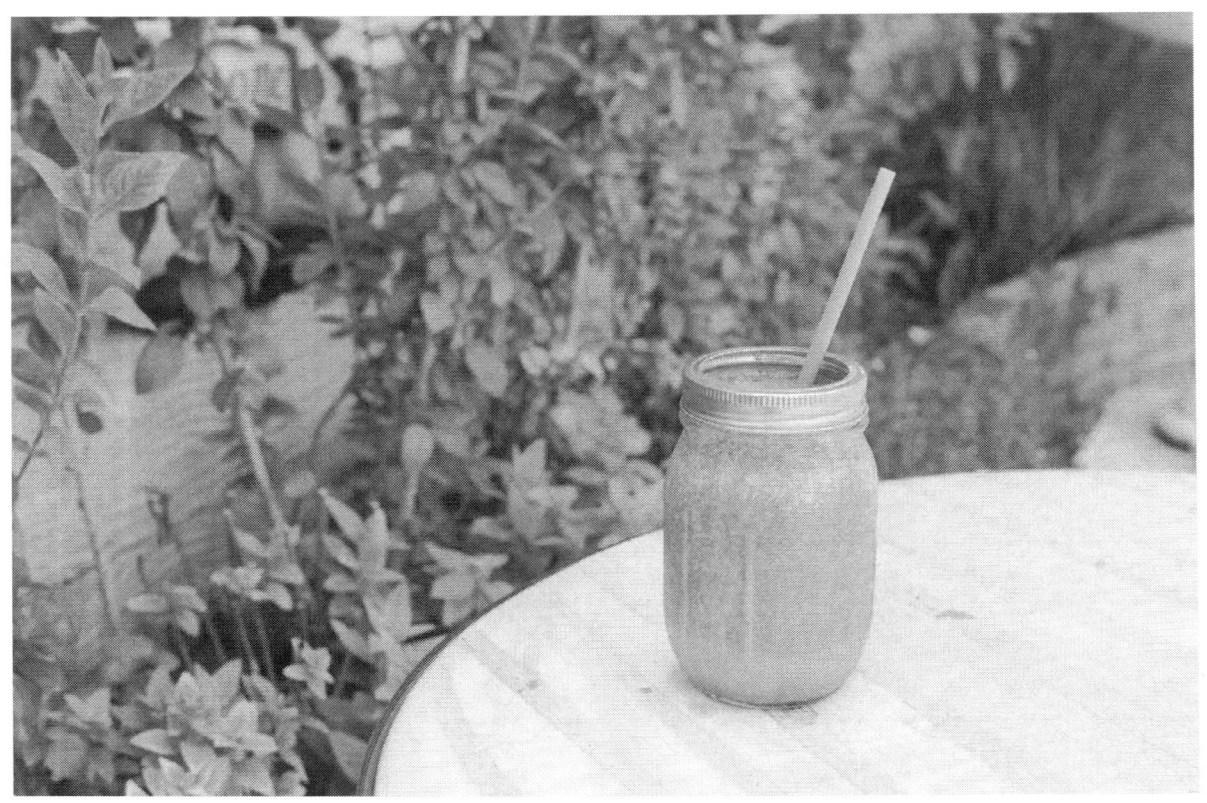

SPICY GINGER CURCUMA SMOOTHIE

1 serving

Ingredients:

200ml of water
½ teaspoon of hemp or linseed oil
¼ lemon
15g of ginger
5ml rice syrup

½ teaspoon of curcuma powder
Cayenne pepper

Preparation:

Put oil, lemon, ginger and the rice syrup along with some water into the mix pot. Then mix at stage 8 for half a minute. Add some more water and mix for 10 seconds at stage 6. Then pour the juice through the sieve insert. Ready to serve!

KCAL	PRO	CAR	FAT
13	1g	2g	0g

FAT BURNER SMOOTHIE

1 serving

Ingredients:

120ml grapefruit juice

100g of organic salad cucumber with shell

10g of ginger

5 basil leaves

2 teaspoon wheatgrass or barley grass

1 teaspoon of cinnamon

1 pinch of chilli, curcuma and pepper

Preparation:

Put the ginger into the mix pot. Then Add all the remaining ingredients and mix for 1 minute at stage 10. If necessary add some water.

Nutritional values per 100ml:

KCAL	PRO	CAR	FAT
71	1g	14g	0g

Smoothies

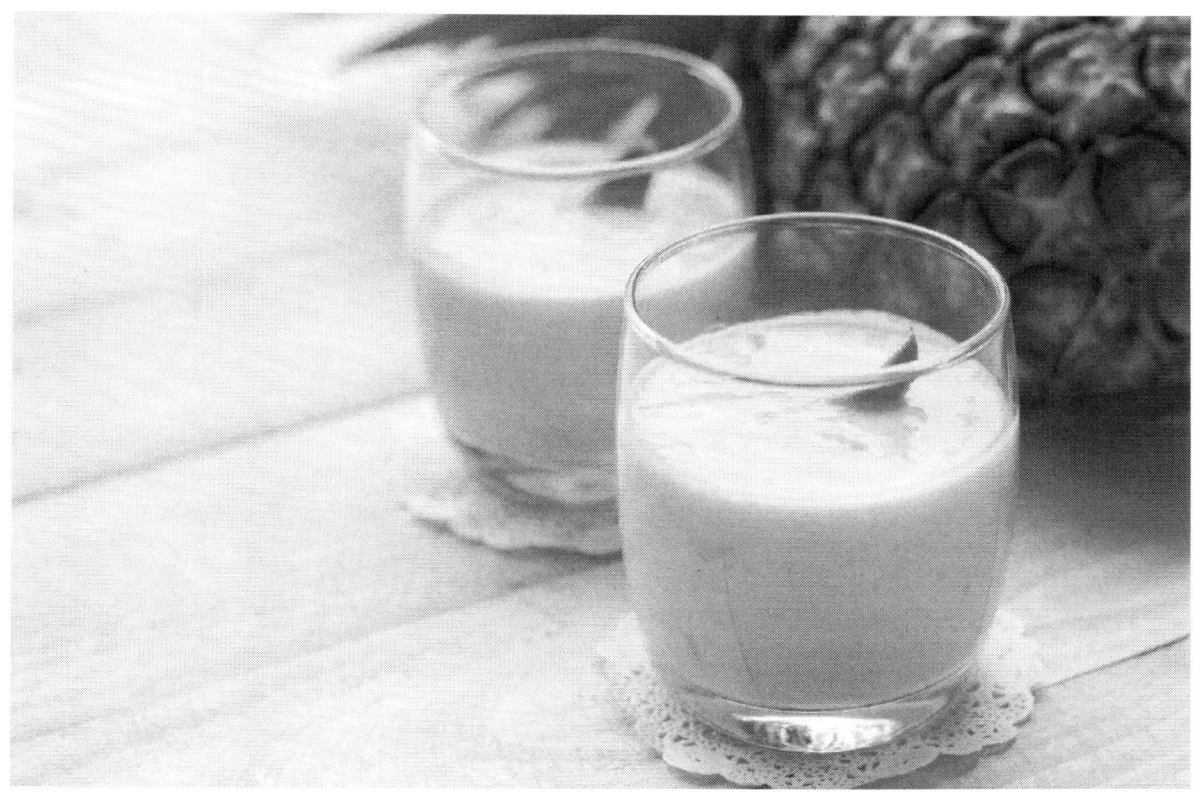

CITRUS AVOCADO SMOOTHIE

2 servings

Ingredients:

100g pineapple

2 oranges

½ avocado

¼ lemon

2 stalks of lemon balm

1 stalk of lemon thyme

Ice cubes

Preparation:
Peel the pineapple and dice it. Wash the oranges well and rub off the peel. Squeeze out the oranges and add the juice. Cut the avocado into halfes and remove the fruit pulp. Squeeze out the lemon, wash the herbs and remove leaves. Add all ingredients together with ice cubes to the mix pot and mix it smooth for 10 seconds at stage 10.

KCAL	PRO	CAR	FAT
148	2g	15g	8g

COCOS SMOOTHIE WITH CARROTS

2 servings

Ingredients:

60g coconut rasp

400ml carrot juice

40ml coconut milk

60g whole milk yoghurt

½ red chilli peppers

1 stalk of coriander

Ice cubes

Preparation:

Put the coconut into the mix pot and roast it without adding fat at stage 2 (100°C), left running mode for 30 seconds. Decant it and let it cool down. Wash the coriander and remove the leaves. Add the chilli peppers, carrot juice, coconut milk and yogurt to the mixing pot. Mix at stage 10 for 8 seconds until it is smooth. Fill it into two glasses and garnish with coriander leaves and coconut chips.

KCAL	PRO	CAR	FAT
320	6g	15g	26g

Smoothies

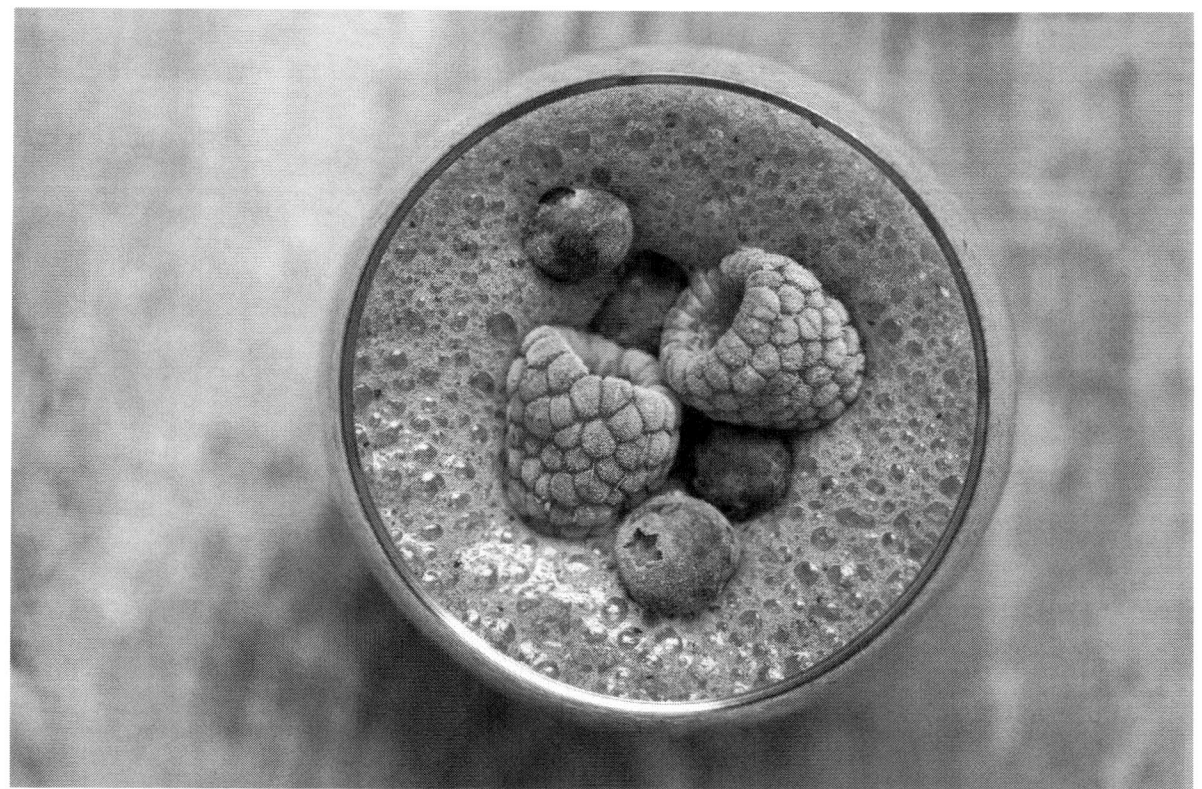

BERRY SHAKE

2 servings

Ingredients:

250ml kefir

1 banana

1 handful of blueberries

3 slices of pineapple

50ml Ananassaft

1 small piece of ginger

Preparation:

Peel the Pineapple and dice it. Then pour all the ingredients into the mix pot and puree for 35 seconds at stage 8.

KCAL	PRO	CAR	FAT
224	0g	24g	0g

Smoothies

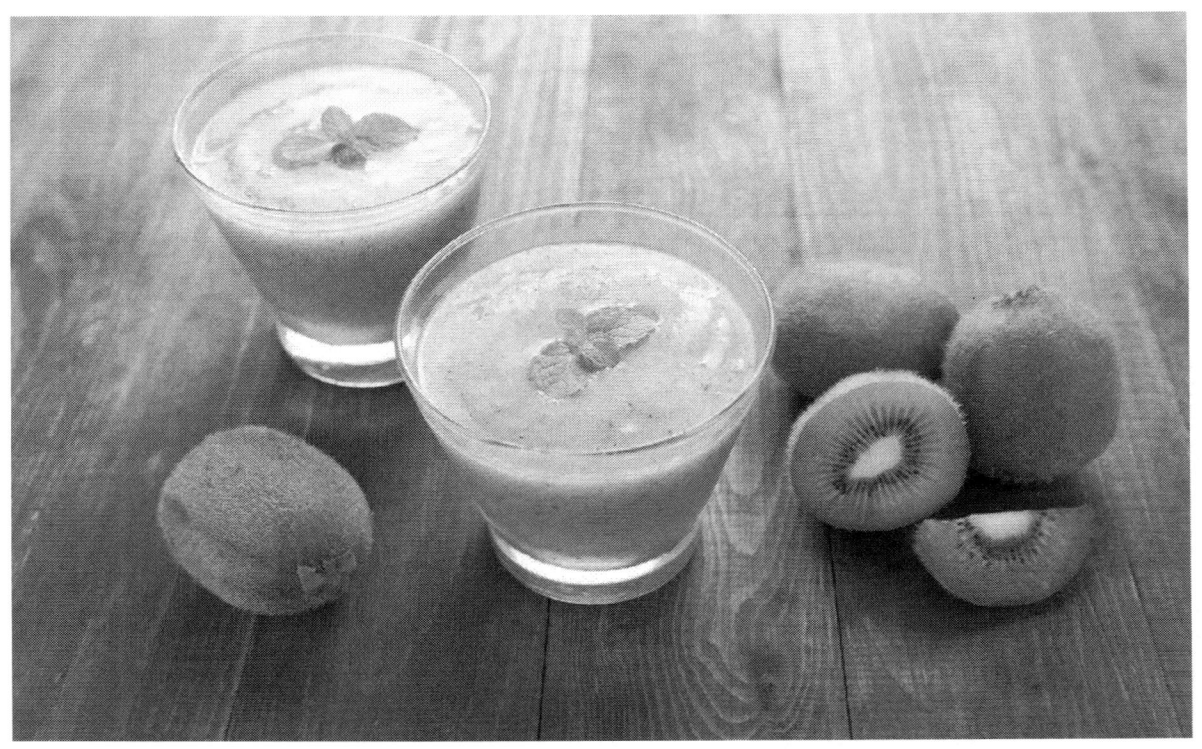

KIWI ALMOND MILK SHAKE

2 servings

Ingredients:

400ml almond milk

3 kiwis

2 teaspoons of Xucker

Vanilla flavour

Preparation:

Peel the kiwi, then pour all the ingredients into the mixing pot and finely mince them at stage 8 for 35 seconds.

KCAL	PRO	CAR	FAT
89	0g	9g	0g

Smoothies

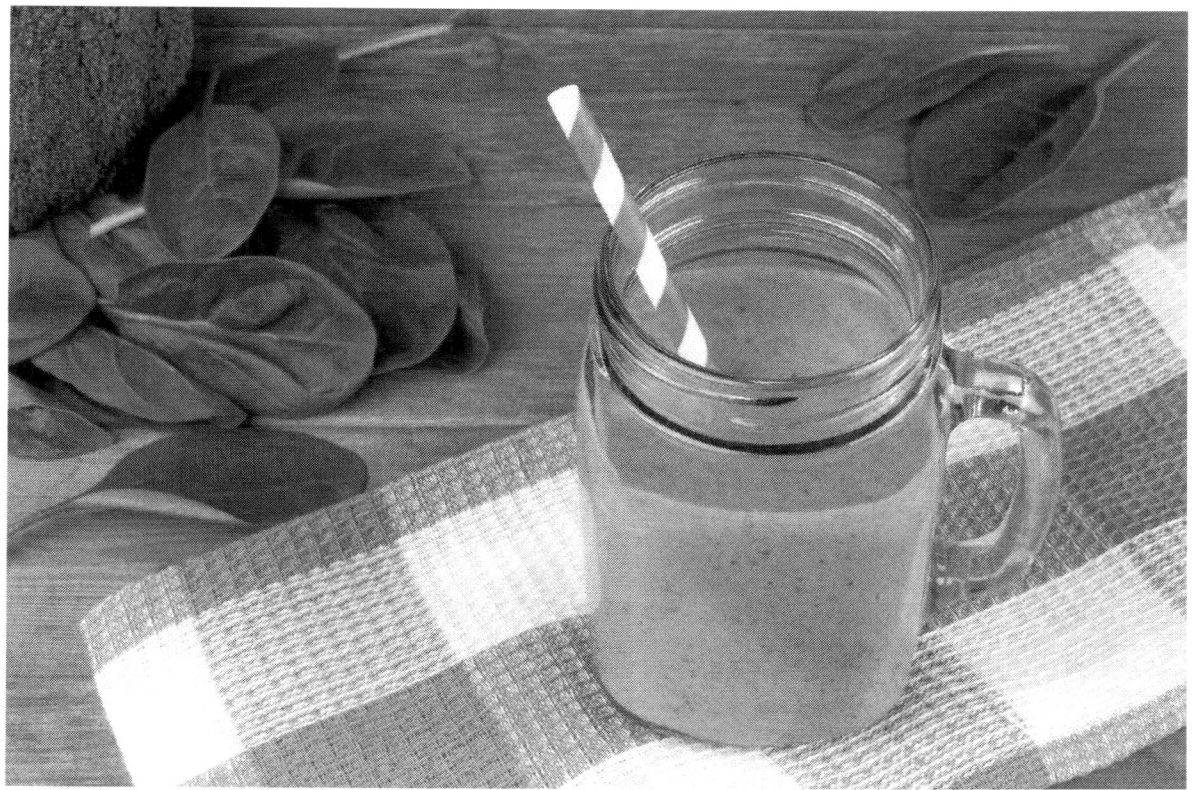

LETTUCE CUCUMBER SMOOTHIE

2 servings

Ingredients:

4 limes

4 cucumbers

4 apples (green)

4 kiwis

1 handful of field salad

Preparation:

Squeeze out the lime. Then wash the cucumbers and cut them into pieces. Wash the apples and remove the cores. Wash the lettuce and clean. Put it into the mixing pot. Stir for 35 seconds at stage 8. Serve with ice cubes.

KCAL	PRO	CAR	FAT
185	0g	22g	0g

Smoothies

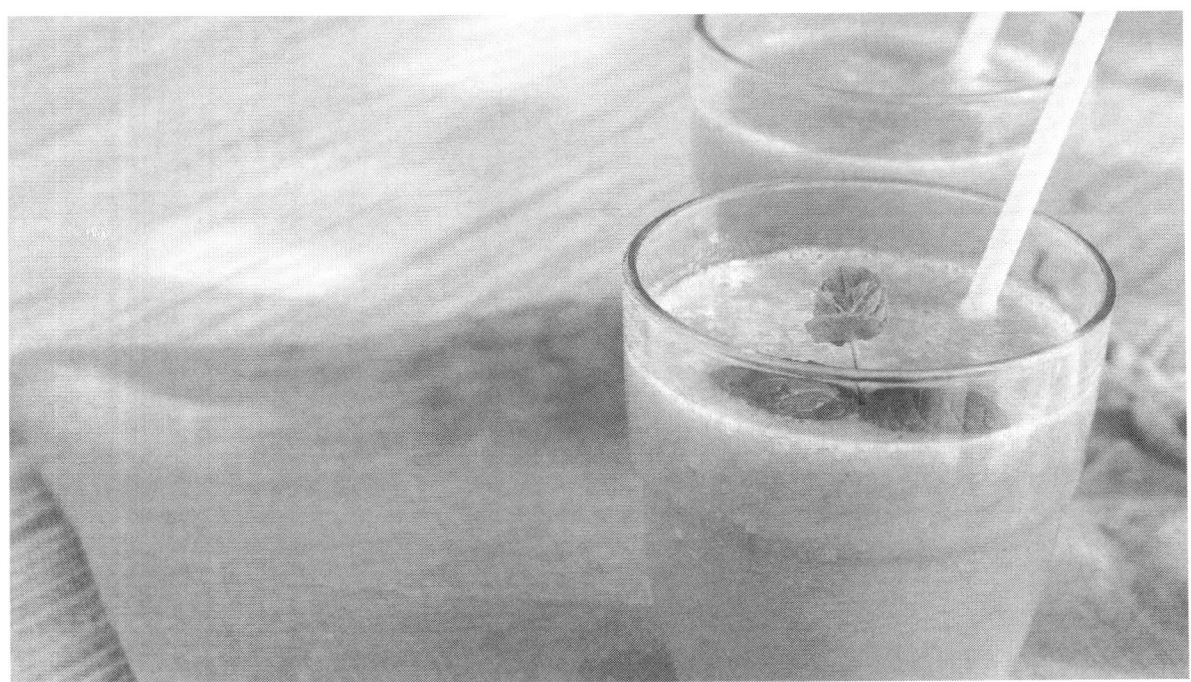

NECTARINE ORANGE SMOOTHIE

2 servings

Ingredients:

2 oranges

2 nectarines

300ml almond milk

1 ½ teaspoon brownhirsemehl

1 tablespoon almonds (ground)

Stevia powder

Preparation:

Peel the orange and halve it, then peel off the pulp and add the remaining ingredients to the cooking machine. Now finely mash for 35 seconds at stage 5-6 and add sweetener as desired.

KCAL	PRO	CAR	FAT
210	0g	27g	1g

Desserts

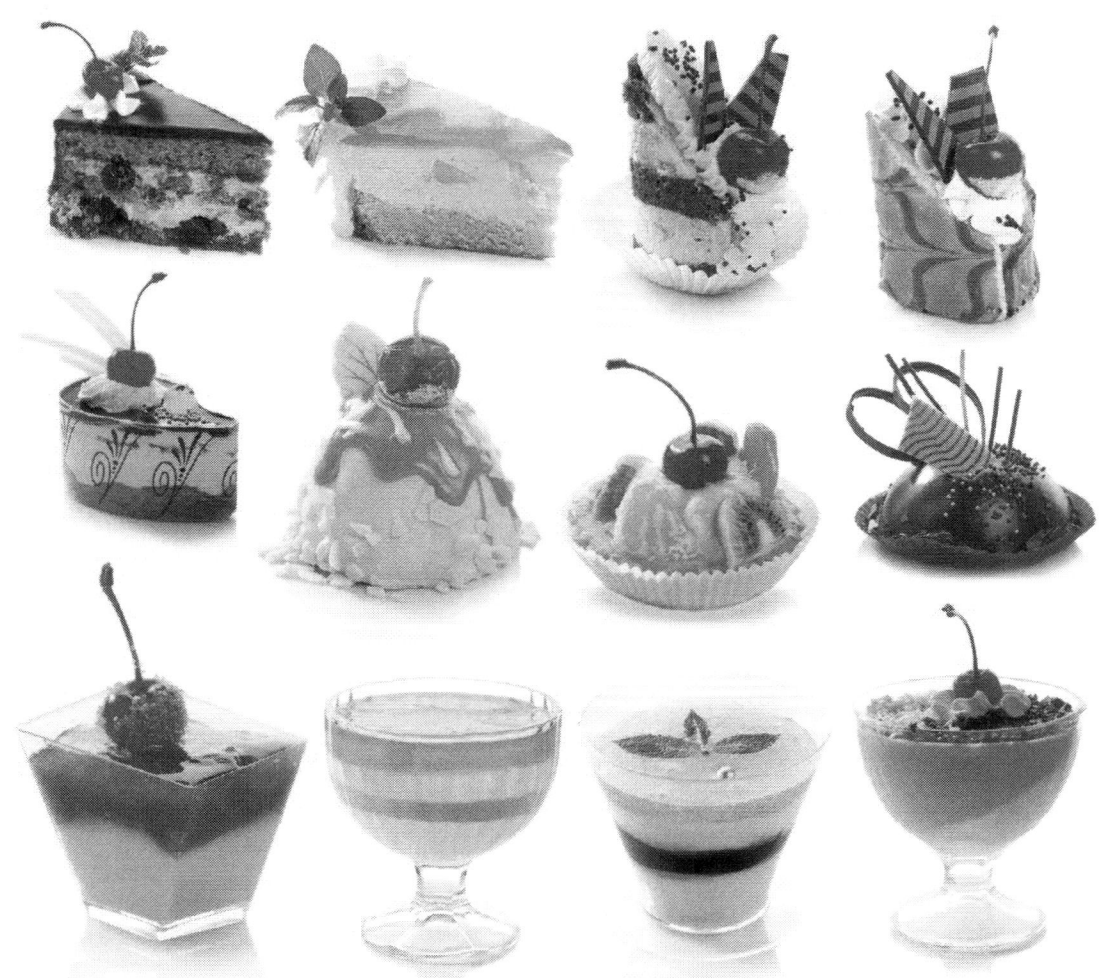

DESSERTS

Raspberry jam 93

Chia coconut pudding 94

Desserts

Chocolate cream 95

Apple cinnamon cream 96

Tiramisu 97

Desserts

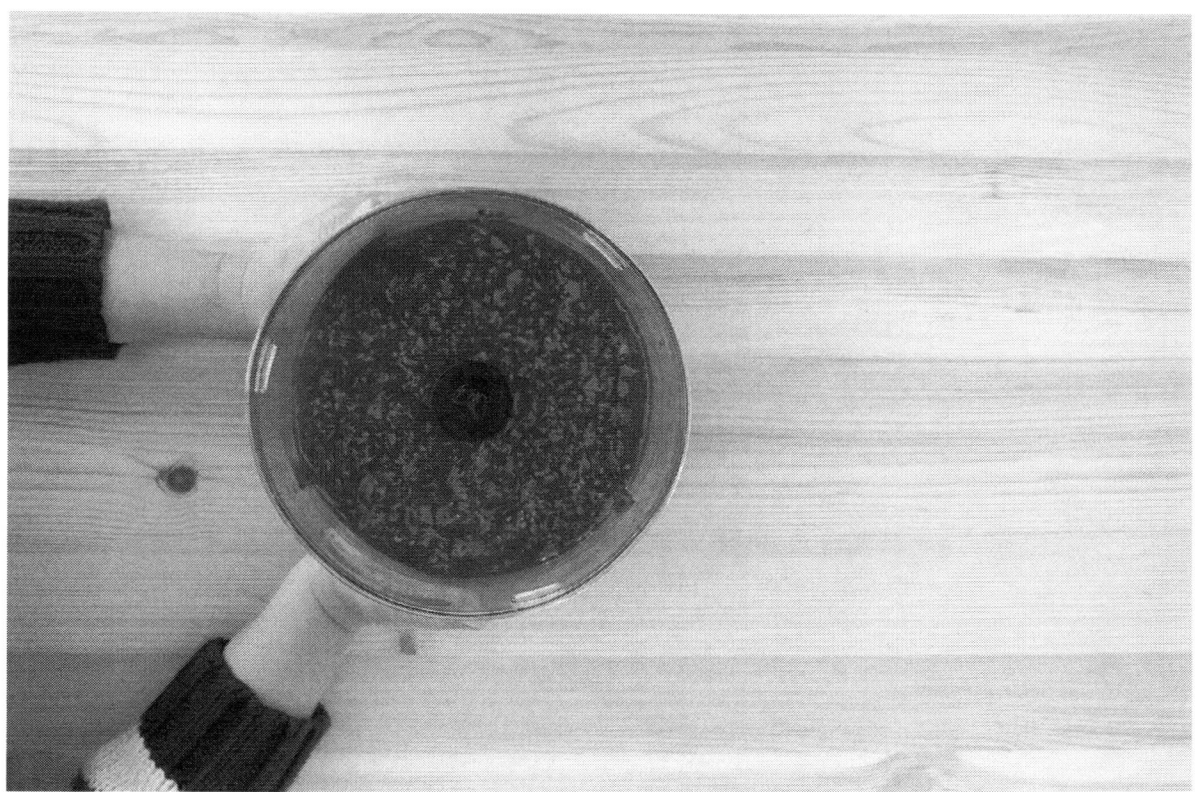

RASPBERRY JAM

2 servings

Ingredients:

200g raspberries

6 tablespoons chia seeds

300ml coconut milk

4 teaspoons coconut

2 teaspoons agave juice

Preparation:

Pour all the ingredients into the mixing pot and mix for 8 seconds at level 4. Fill into jars and allow to swell for 30 minutes.

KCAL	PRO	CAR	FAT
174	0g	11g	0g

Desserts

CHIA COCONUT PUDDING

2 servings

Ingredients:

150g yoghurt

200ml coconut milk

4 teaspoons of chia seeds

2 kiwi

Xucker

Preparation:

Combine the chia seeds with the coconut milk and mix for 1 minute. Leave to simmer overnight and add the jelly-like mass and yoghurt to the mixing pot. Stir for 5 seconds at level 3 and place in two jars. Peel the kiwi and place in the mixing pot. For 7 minutes at level 6 puree and then with Xucker sweet as desired and over the Chia yogurt give.

Nutritional values per 100g:

KCAL	PRO	CAR	FAT
128	0g	9g	0g

Desserts

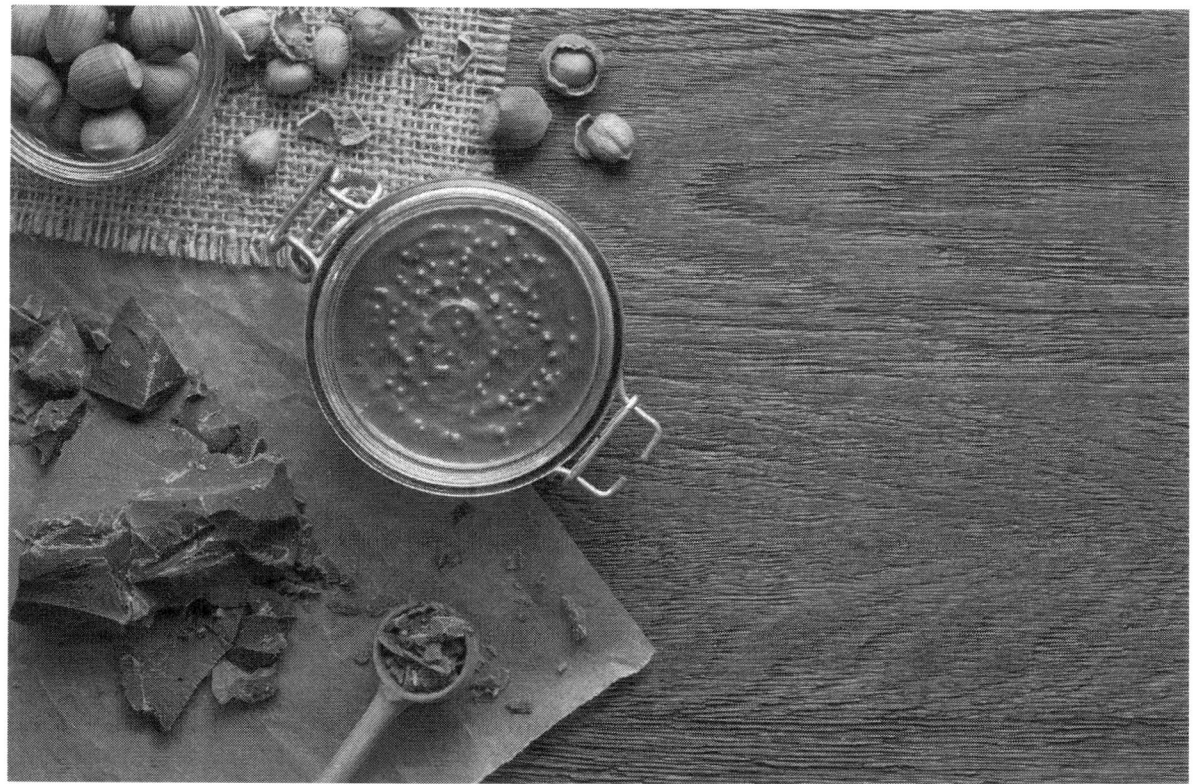

CHOCOLATE CREAM

2 servings

Ingredients:

160ml cream

80g dark chocolate

2 candied gingers

Preparation:

Put the ginger and chocolate in pieces in the mix pot. Crush for 12 seconds at level 6-7 and add the cream. Set to 8 for 8 seconds. Pour into a glass bowl and serve.

KCAL	PRO	CAR	FAT
378	0g	18g	0g

Desserts

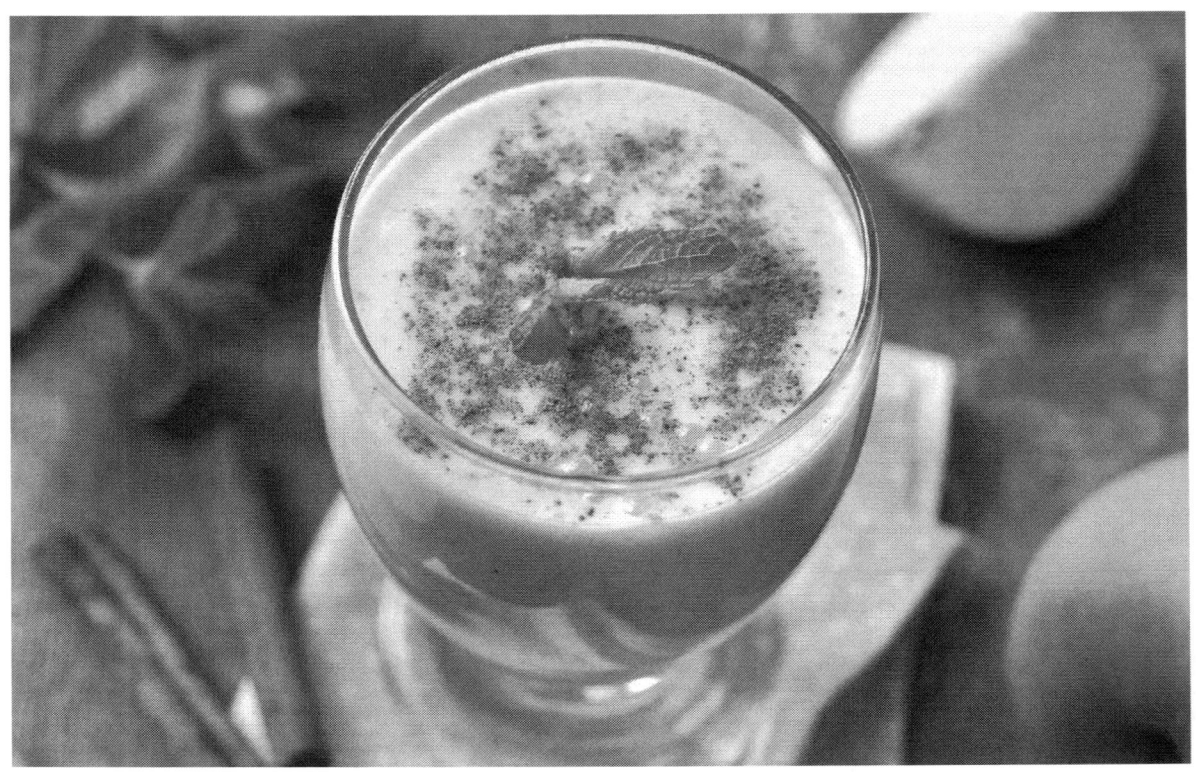

APPLE CINNAMON CREAM

2 servings

Ingredients:

2 apples

1 lime

100g of double cream cheese

100g yoghurt

Cinnamon

Xucker

Preparation:

Peel the apples and place them into the mixing pot. Crush for 3 seconds at stage 4. Add lemon juice, fresh cheese and cinnamon and stir for 2 seconds at stage 2. Add Xucker according to your taste.

KCAL	PRO	CAR	FAT
245	0g	18g	0g

Desserts

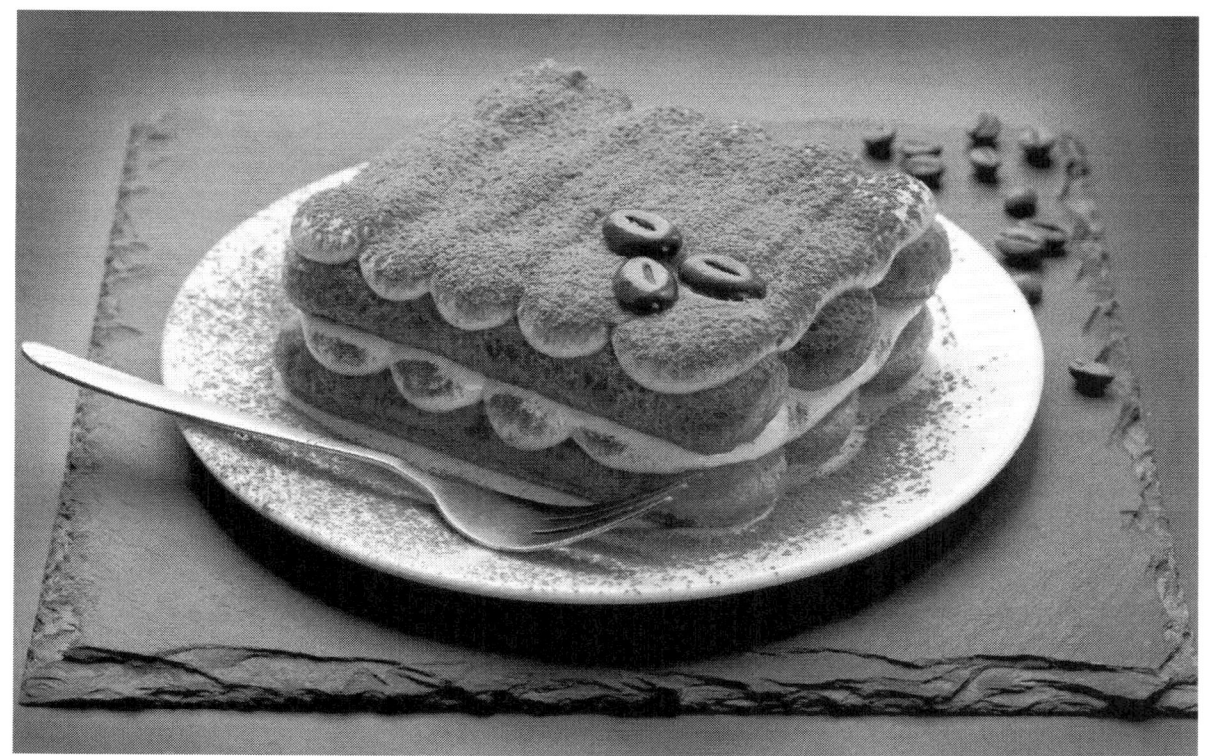

TIRAMISU

4 servings

Ingredients:

60g ground almonds

3 eggs

2 egg yolks

300g mascarpone

2 teaspoons of Xucker

80ml coffee

Amaretto syrup

Cocoa for garnishing

Desserts

Preparation:

Separate the eggs and put the egg whites into the mix pot. Whip at stage 4 and then decant into a separate bowl. Preheat oven to 180 °C. Mix the egg yolks, Xucker and the almonds together. Then fold in gently the whipped egg whites. Now place the mass on a baking sheet and bake it for 20 minutes at 180 degrees in the preheated oven. Then put the mascarpone, egg yolk and Xucker into the mix pot and stir for 1 minute at level 4.

Season with Amaretto according to taste. When the dough is done let it cool down and then cut it into small pieces. Now put the pieces out to a layer on the bottom of a mold and soak it with some coffee. Then spread half of the mascarpone cream evenly over it. Proceed in the same way with the next layer and again soak it with coffee. Then spread out the remaining mascarpone cream. Leave it in the fridge overnight. Sprinkle some cocoa powder over the tiramisu before serving.

KCAL	PRO	CAR	FAT
320	0g	4g	2g

Snacks

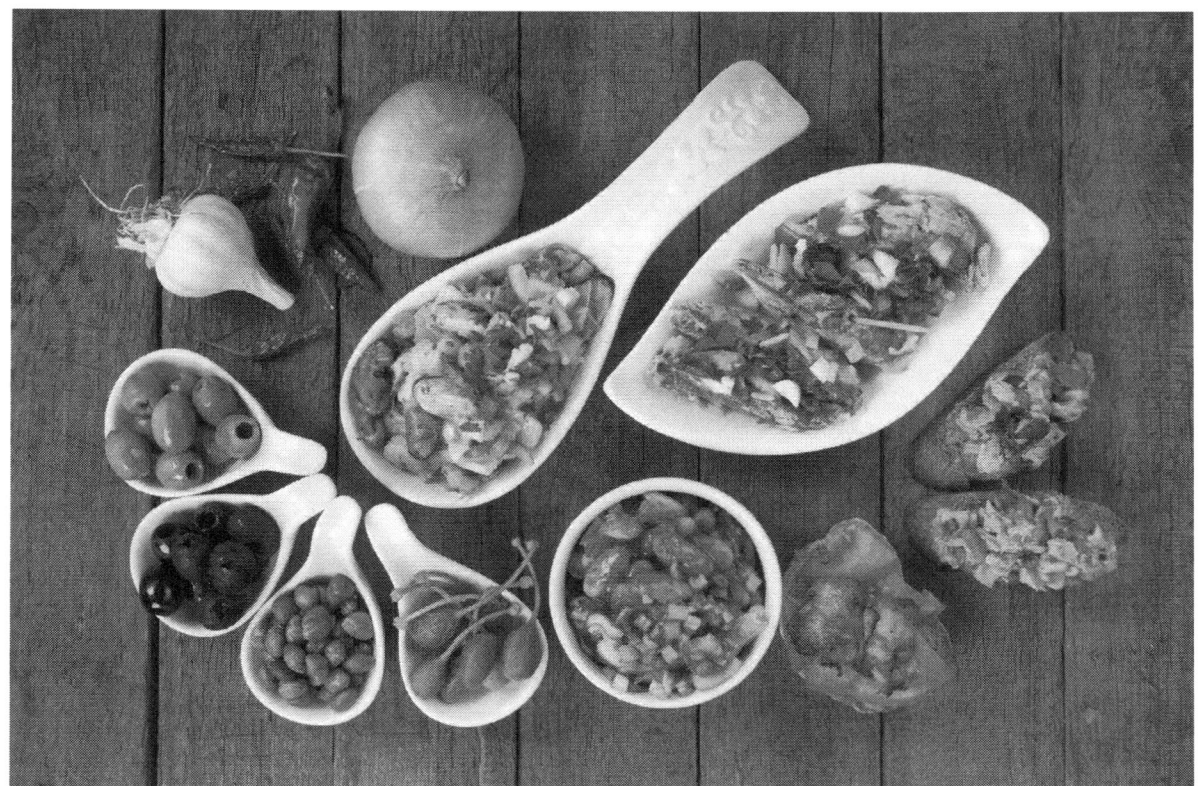

SNACKS

Chocolate cake..100

Nut bars..101

Raffaelo 102

Chia pudding 103

Coconut yogurt with melon..............................104

Snacks

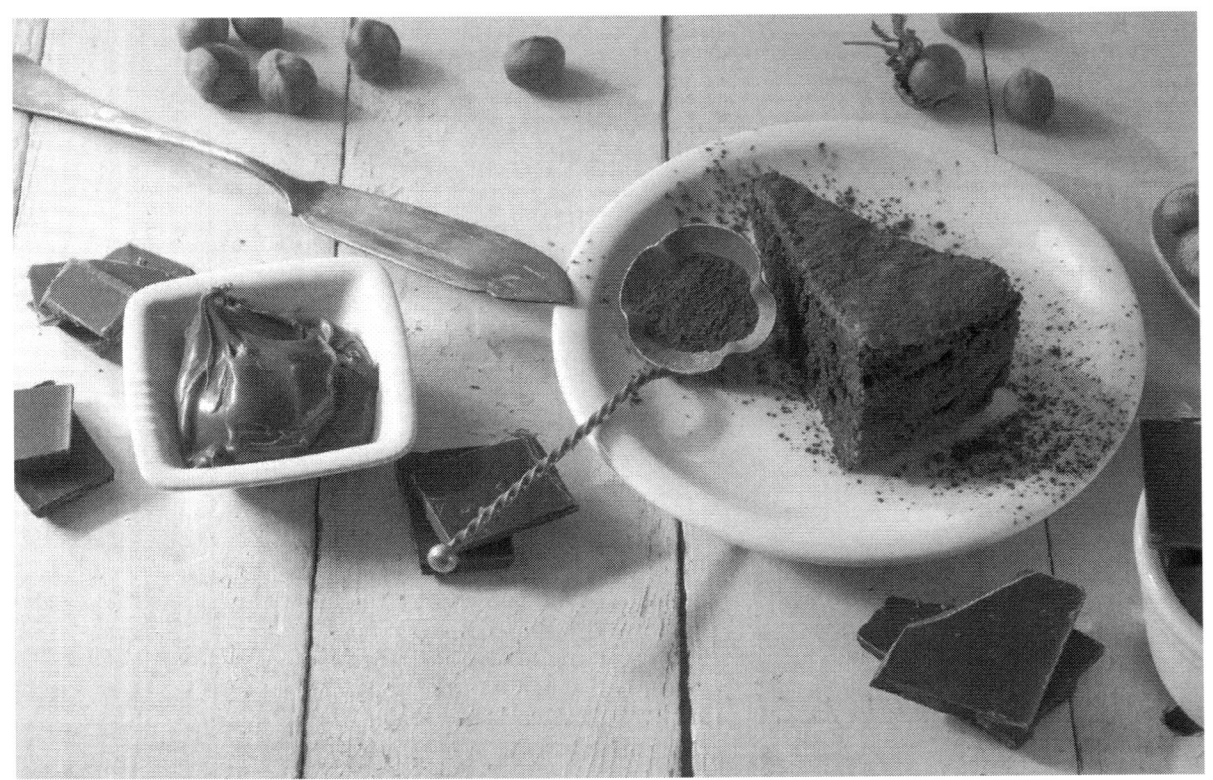

CHOCOLATE CAKE

For 10 pieces

Ingredients:

200g of dark chocolate (55%)

130g butter

150g Erythritol or Xucker

90g almond flour

5 eggs

8 small pieces of chocolate

Preparation:

Shred the chocolate for 10 seconds at stage 10. Add butter and melt it at stage 1 for 4 minutes. Add eggs, Xucker, the almond flour and stir at stage 4 for 1 minute. Fill the dough in the muffin forms, until they are filled completely. Bake it for 12 minutes at stage 8 and enjoy fresh.

KCAL	PRO	CAR	FAT
295	25g	17g	9g

NUT BARS

Snacks

For 20 pieces

Ingredients:

60g coconut chips

60g pumpkin seeds

60g sunflower seeds

60g walnuts

40g hazelnuts

20g sesame

6 stoned dates

40g cocoa

2 tsp cinnamon

6 teaspoons of coconut milk

3 teaspoons of almond puree

Preparation:

Put pumpkin seeds, coconut flakes, sunflower seeds, walnuts, dates and the hazelnuts in the cooking machine and shred for 10 seconds at stage 5-6. Add cocoa, cinnamon, sesame, almonds and the coconut milk and mix for 10 seconds at stage 3. Preheat oven to 100°C. Then grease a baking pan with coconut oil and fill in the nut mass. Bake it in the preheated oven for 50 minutes. Take it out and let it cool down completely. Then cut the hazelnut mass into bars.

KCAL	PRO	CAR	FAT
104	4g	3g	6g

Snacks

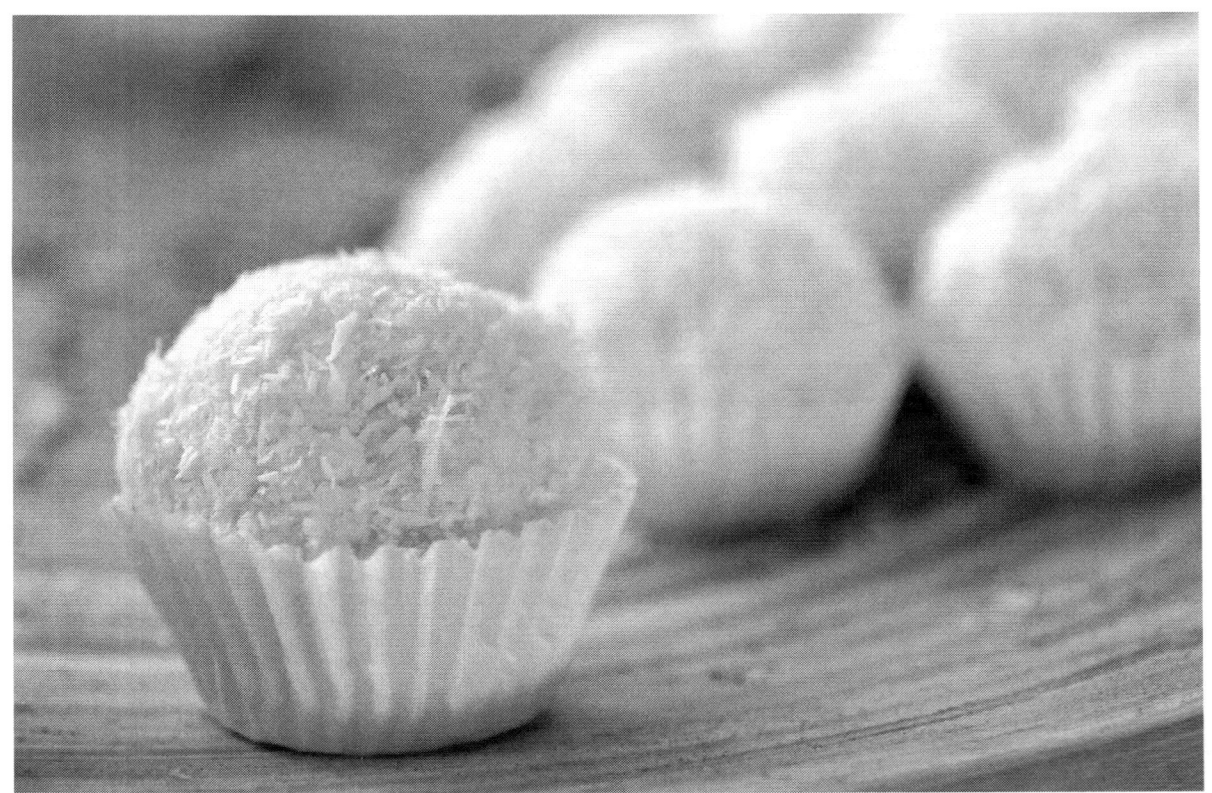

RAFFAELO

For 20 pieces

Ingredients:

400g of lean starch

90g of ground almonds

10 almonds

35g coconut flakes

45g of protein powder

Sweetener

Preparation:

Put all the ingredients into the mixing pot and mix them thoroughly. Then form the dough to about 10 scoops. Roll the balls through coconut flakes till they are covered all around. Put an almond on top of each and leave them in the refrigerator for 4 hours.

KCAL	PRO	CAR	FAT
30	0g	5g	0g

Snacks

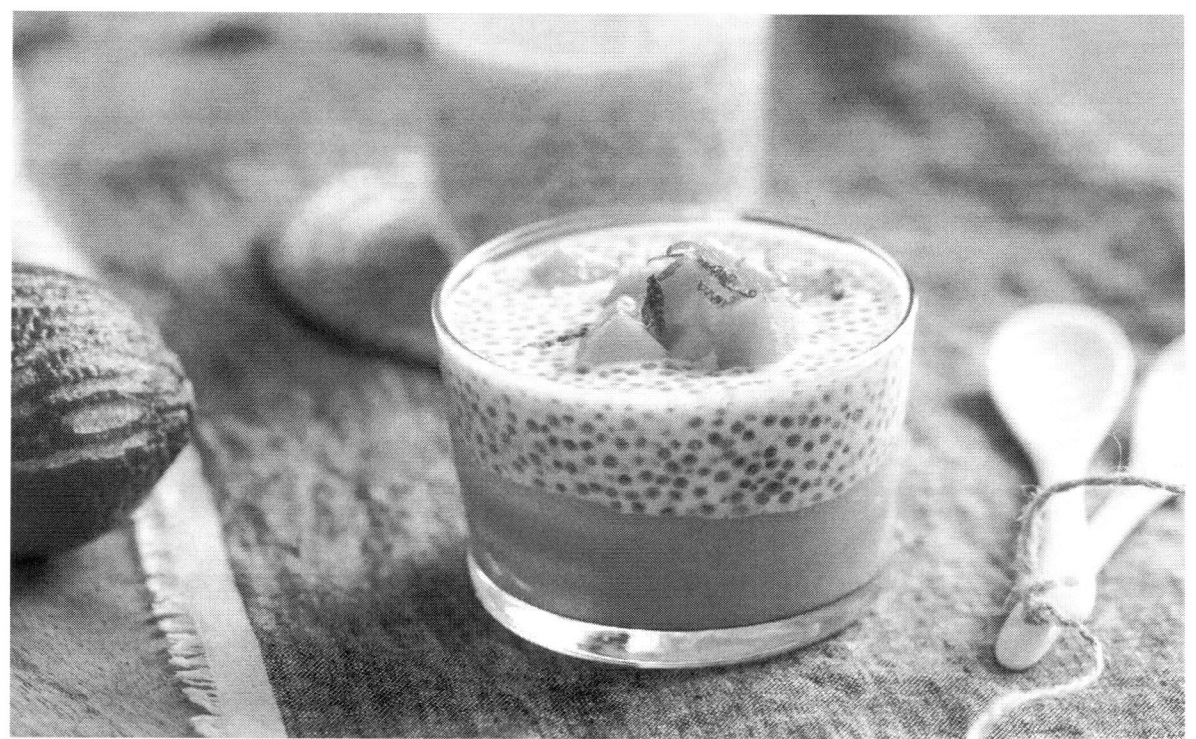

CHIA PUDDING

2 servings

Ingredients:

½ mango

2 teaspoons of chia seeds

200ml almond milk

60g raspberries

Preparation:
Put the chia seeds in a bowl and pour in the almond milk. Stir by hand for about 1 minute. Let the chia seeds swell overnight. Peel the mango and cut it into coarse pieces. Then put it into the mix pot and puree for 7 seconds at stage 5. Then put the chia pudding into 2 glasses and pour the mango purée over it. Garnish with raspberries.

KCAL	PRO	CAR	FAT
85	0g	9g	0g

Snacks

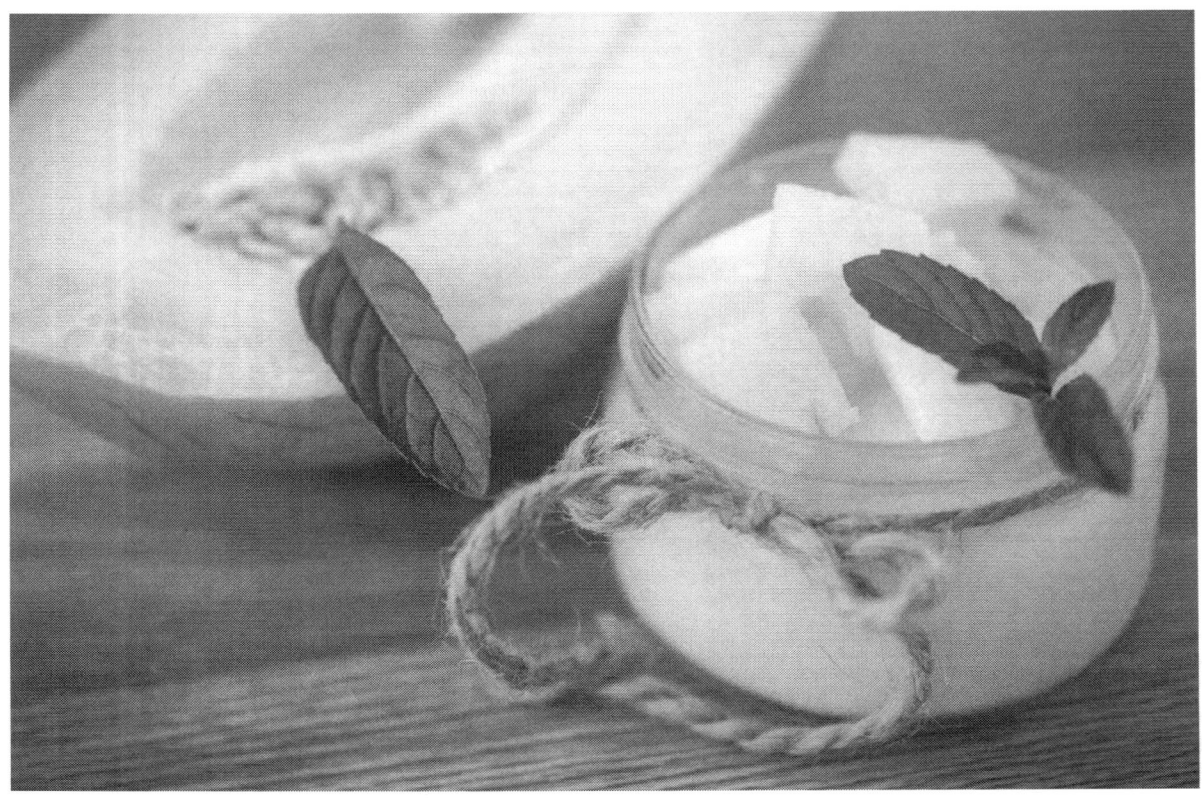

COCONUT YOGURT WITH MELON

2 servings

Ingredients:

250g honey melon

125g curd

150g yoghurt

1 teaspoon of coconut rasps

1 stalk of mint

½ lemon

1 teaspoon of maple syrup

Preparation:

Roast the coconut rasps in a coated pan without adding grease and then let them cool down. Squeeze the lemon and pour the juice into the mix pot. Add the curd, the maple syrup and the yoghurt and then stir for 15 seconds at stage 3. Add the roasted coconut rasps and mix for 10 seconds.

Remove the stones from the melon and cut it into small cubes, then mingle with the yogurt. Pluck off the mint leaves from the stalks and wash them, dry well and then cut them into fine strips. Fill the yogurt into small bowls and garnish with mint.

Nutritional values per 100g:

KCAL	PRO	CAR	FAT
198	3g	16g	1g

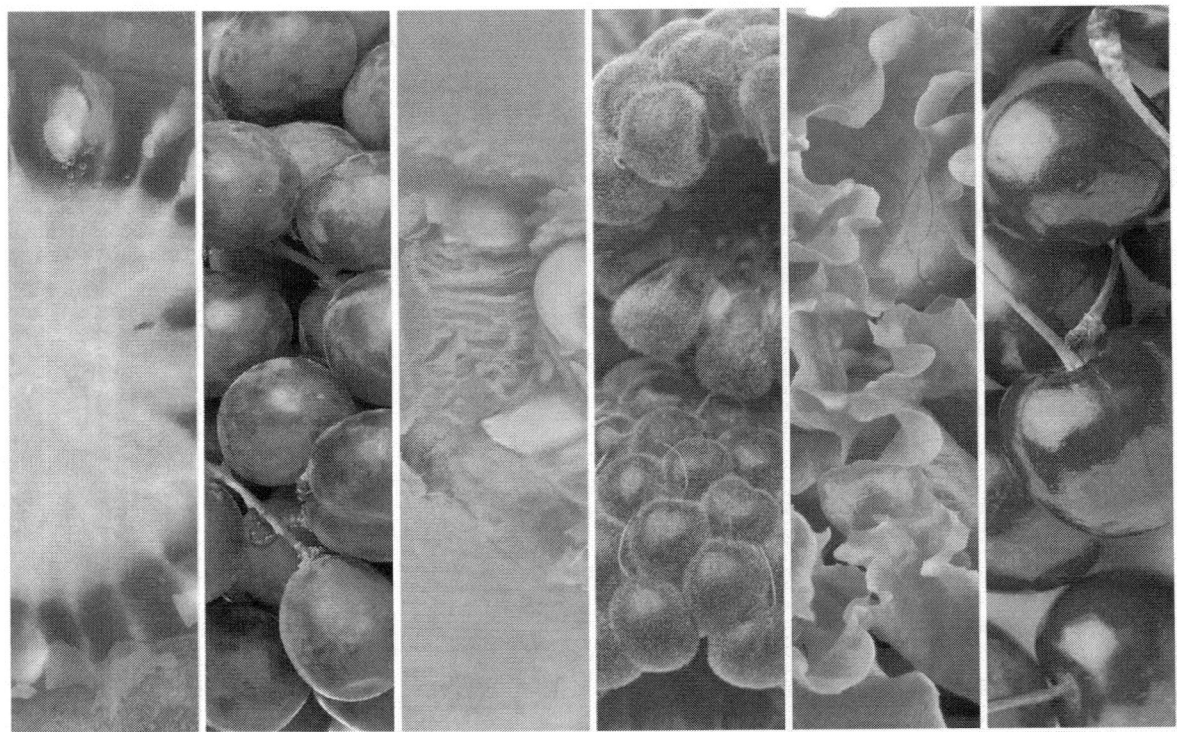

CONCLUDING

Enrich your diet with Low Carb for the cooking machine. You will not only save a lot of time, you will also get used to a healthy diet and do something good for your body and your soul. In addition, you will easily lose weight and provide your whole family with a healthy diet. As a bonus I added my personal 6 sweets and snacks recipes. I hope you will enjoy following the recipes and that I could help you with my advices.

Thank you for choosing my book!

Anna Lange

Bonus

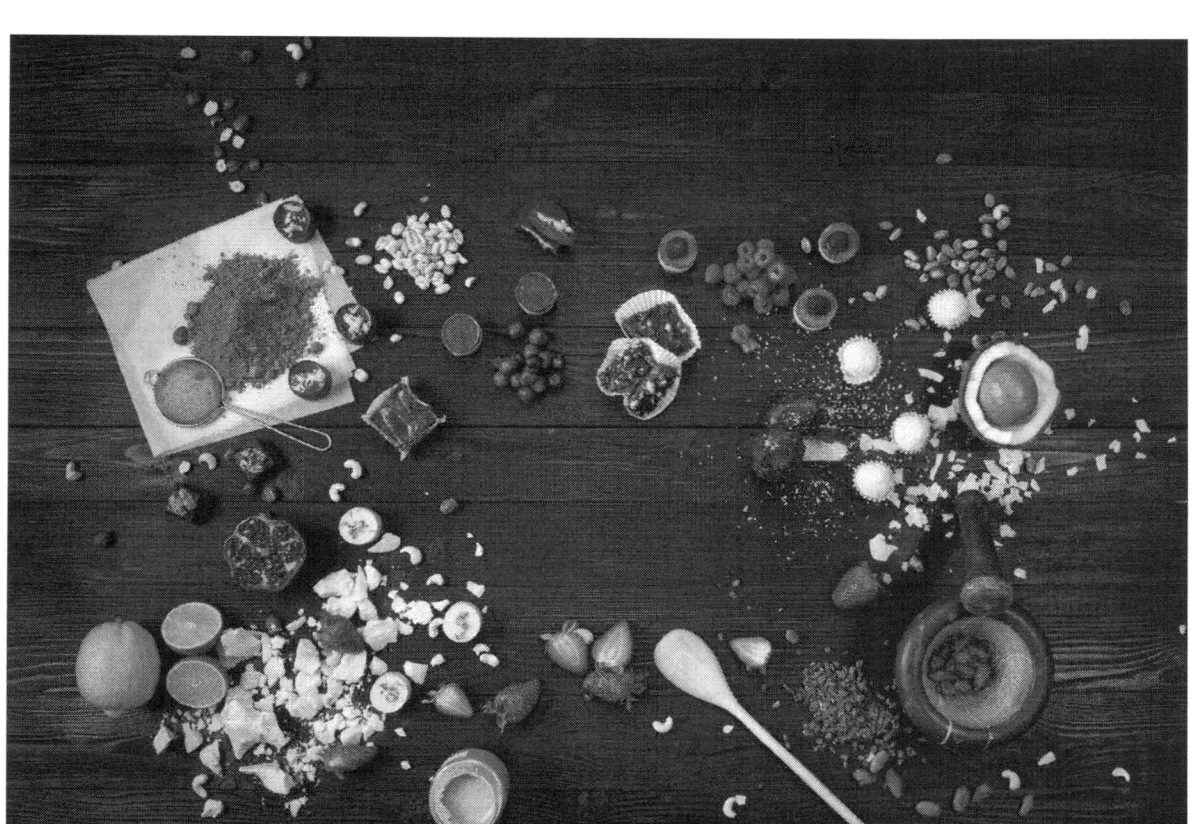

BONUS: MY FAVOURITE 6 SWEET RECIPES

Brownies..109

Strawberry coconut cream..................................111

Apple Pie..112

Coconut Quark..114

Bonus

Strawberry Sorbet 115

Quark Sorbet 116

Bonus

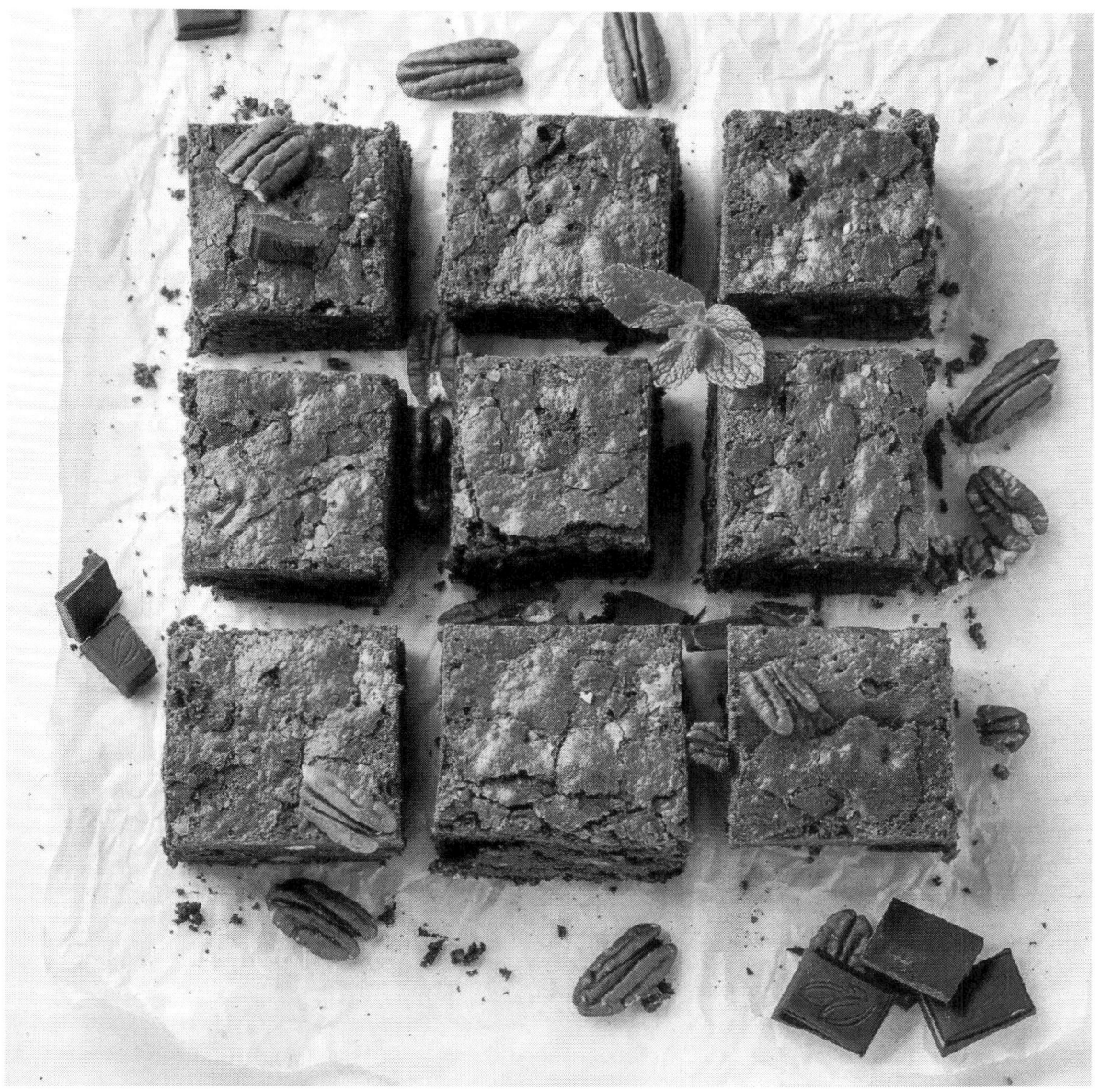

BROWNIES

12 servings

Ingredients:

125g almond flour
3 teaspoons cocoa powder
2 teaspoons linseed
1 teaspoon Baking powder
75g Xucker
50g chocolate with 70% cocoa content
75g margarine
50g almonds
Salt

Preparation:

Place the linseed in a small bowl and pour hot water over. Let it swell for 10 minutes. Then put the almond flour, cocoa powder, baking powder and the Xucker in a bowl. Pour the almonds into the mixing pot and shred them at stage 6 for 3 seconds. Then add chocolate, margarine and some salt and let it melt at stage 2 (80 °C) for about 4 minutes.

Add the almond flour and the linseed in the mixing pot and mix at level 3 for 10 seconds. Preheat oven to 180 degrees with upper and lower heat. Then coat a baking pan with some margarine and fill the dough into it. Put it into the oven and bake it for 30 minutes.

KCAL	PRO	CAR	FAT
110	6g	3g	8g

STRAWBERRY COCONUT CREAM

2 servings

Ingredients:

100g strawberries

100g lean quark

2 tablespoons coconut milk

5 macadamia nuts

2 tablespoons xucker

1 stalk of lemon balm

Preparation:

Put the nuts into the mix pot and shred at stage 5 for 3 seconds. Decant it. Into a separate bowl. Wash the strawberries and chop them at stage 5 for 3 seconds. Add curd, coconut milk, Xucker and nuts and mix at stage 1 for 5 seconds in left running mode. Fill it in 2 dessert bowls and garnish as desired.

KCAL	PRO	CAR	FAT
131	8g	11g	7g

Bonus

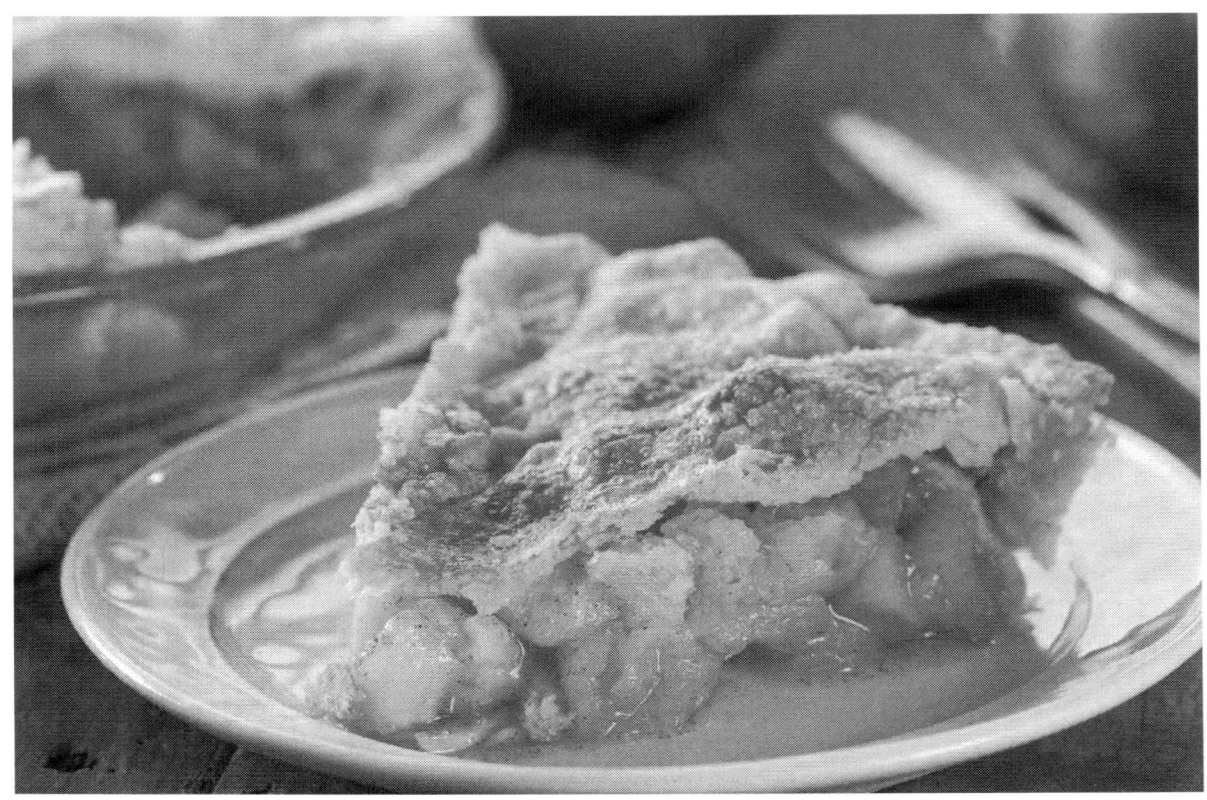

APPLE PIE

4 servings

Ingredients:

100g sour apples

125g almond flour

75g butter

85g Xucker

2 eggs

½ lemon

¼ Pack of baking soda

½ vanilla shake

Cinnamon and salt (as desired)

Preparation:

Squeeze out the lemon and pour the juice in a bowl filled with cold water. Halve the apples and core them, then add them to the mix pot. Crush at 1 stage 6 for 3 seconds. Then put them in the bowl with the lemon water. Add the Xucker, butter, eggs and cinnamon to the mix pot and mix at stage 2 for 5 seconds. Cut the vanilla pod lengthwise, then scrap them out and add them to the mix pod. Add the almond flour, salt and baking powder into the mix pot and then mix at stage 2 for 5 seconds.

Spread the Varoma appplication with baking paper and spread the apples on it. Fill the dough into the mold. Now put the water into the mixing pot, insert the Varoma application and cook for 50 minutes at stage 1. When it is done fill in the dough upside down into a pan and fry for 15 minutes at medium heat.

KCAL	PRO	CAR	FAT
300	17g	8g	21g

Bonus

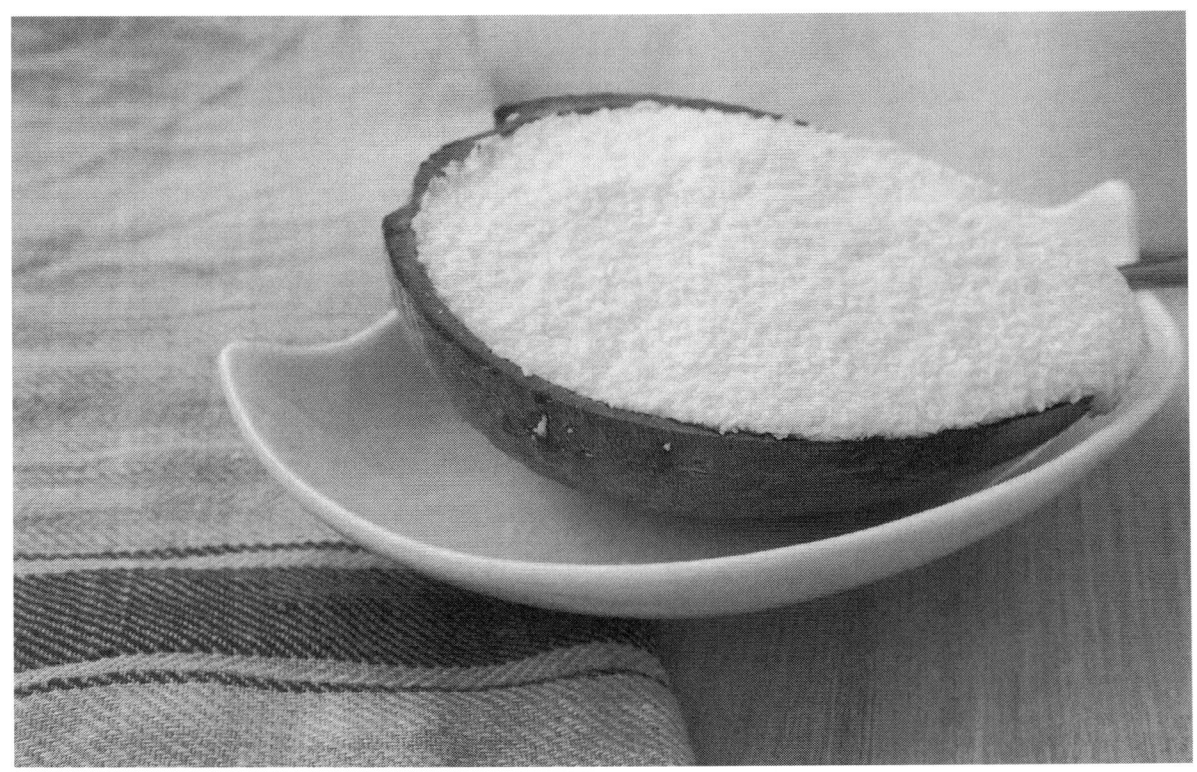

COCONUT QUARK

2 servings

Ingredients:

400g of lean starch

200ml of coconut water

2 teaspoons of protein powder

4 teaspoons of coconut

2 tablespoons Xucker

2 stalks of lemon balm

Preparation:

Pour all the ingredients into the mixing pot and mix them at stage 3 for 10 seconds. Garnish with lemon balm.

KCAL	PRO	CAR	FAT
183	29g	10g	2g

Bonus

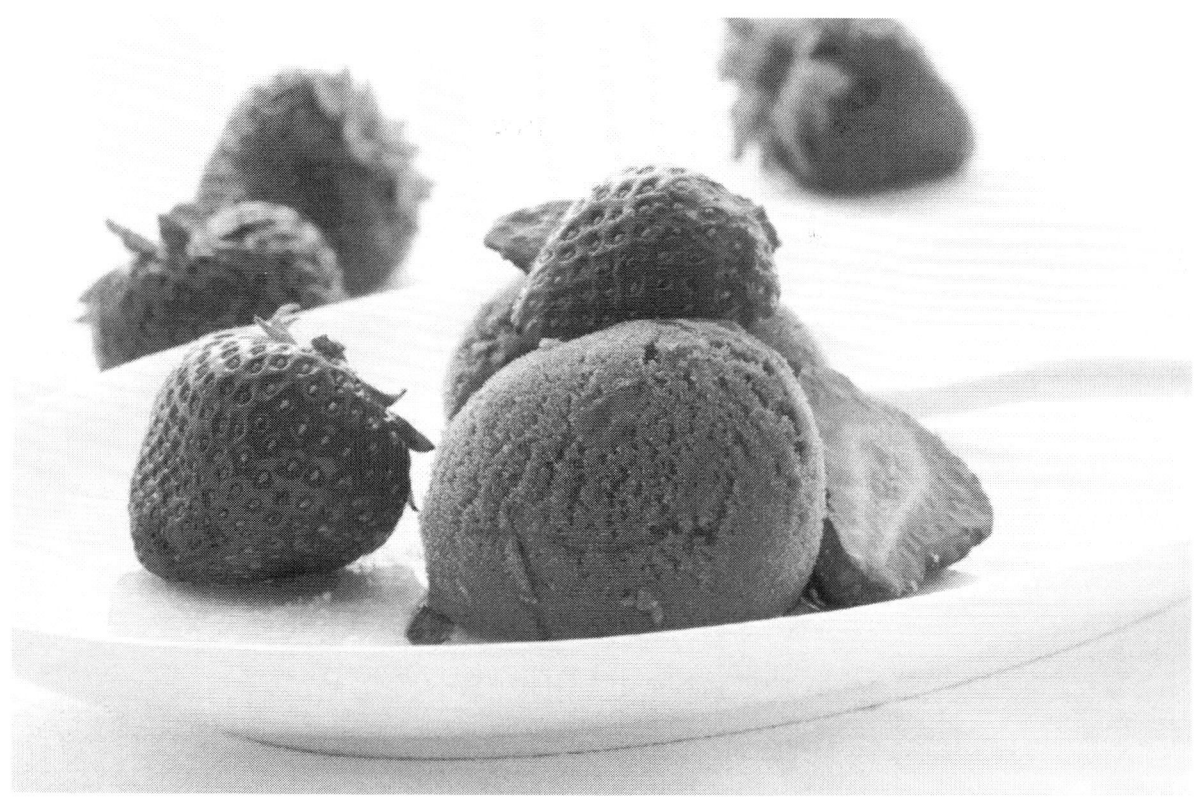

STRAWBERRY SORBET

2 servings

Ingredients:

300g frozen strawberries

60g protein powder

200ml of water

sweetener

Preparation:

Put the protein powder with the water to the mix pot and mix at stage 5 for 3 seconds. Add fruits and sweetener and puree at stage 10 for 5 seconds. Fill it in a form and leave it in a freezer for at least 1 hour.

KCAL	PRO	CAR	FAT
105	26g	12g	2g

Bonus

QUARK SORBET

2 servings

Ingredients:

300g of low fat curd

60g of protein powder (vanilla flavor)

200ml water

Sweetener

2 handful of ice cubes

Preparation:

Put the protein powder and the water into the mix pot and then mix for 3 seconds at stage 5. Then add curd, ice cubes and the sweetener and puree at stage 10 for 5 seconds. Fill it into a mold and leave it in the freezer for at least 1 hour.

KCAL	PRO	CAR	FAT
105	26g	12g	2g

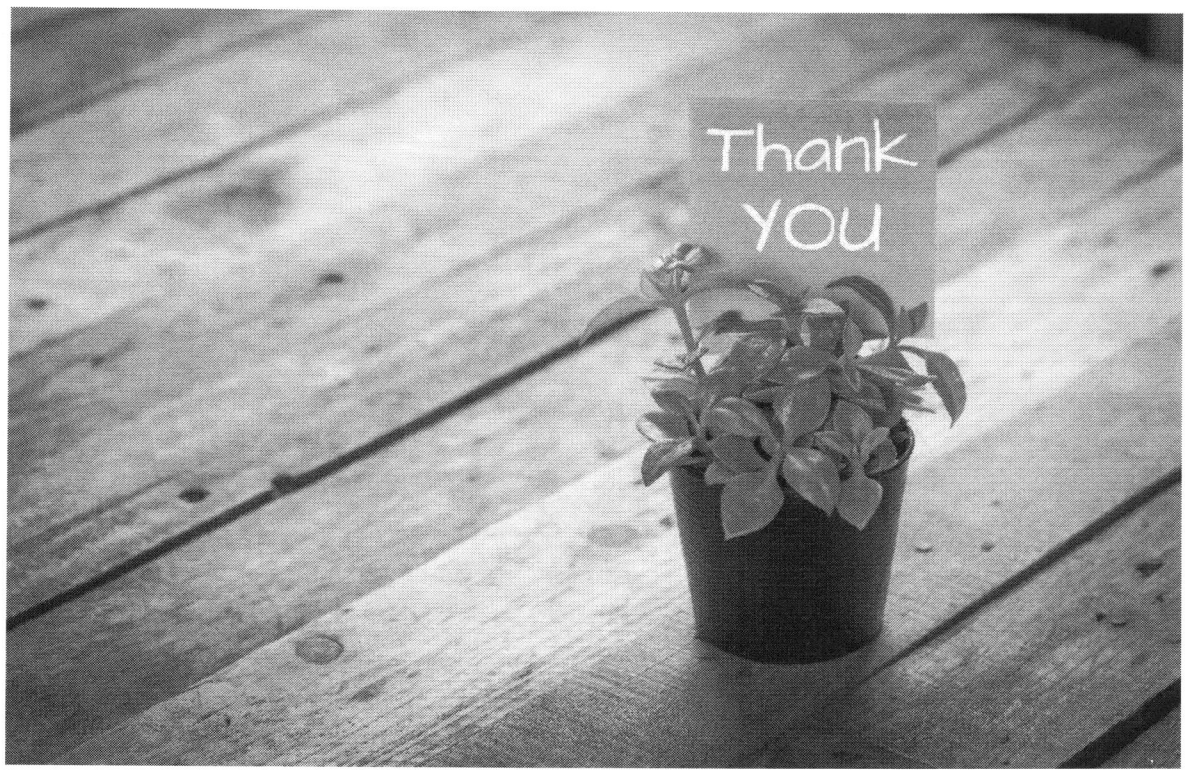

THANK YOU!

I would like to thank you again for buying my book. There are dozens of books, but you decided to get mine. Therefore, a big Thank You for downloading it and reading it to the end.

I would really appreciate to get a review from you <u>on Amazon</u>. A feedback helps me to improve my next books and to help more people with their weight and healthy lifestyle. So if you liked this book, please let me know!

Printed in Great Britain
by Amazon